Contemporary Diagnosis and Management of

Male Erectile Dysfunction®

Tom F. Lue, MD
Professor of Urology
University of California School of Medicine

San Francisco, California

Second Edition

Published by
Handbooks in Health Care Co.,
Newtown, Pennsylvania, USA

International Standard Book Number: 1-931981-44-2

Library of Congress Catalog Card Number: 2004117018

Table of Contents

The author wishes to thank his patients and colleagues for their encouragement and suggestions, which gave birth to many of the new ideas and innovations in this book. The following is a letter from a patient whose identity has been withheld.

Dear Dr. Lue,

I want to take a moment to thank you for giving me the opportunity to change my life. As a result of my accident, I was unable to gain an erection for 14 years. Because of your research and subsequent treatment program, I can now have normal sexual relations on a regular basis.

In some respects, it is actually better than normal because of the increase in staying power.

In the past I felt insecure and socially alienated by my problem. Thanks to you, I have regained my self-confidence. This has had a positive impact on all aspects of my life.

My self-image has improved, my level of stress is reduced and, consequently, my attitude towards life in general is markedly enhanced.

It is good once again to feel like a man.

Best regards,

Chapter 1

Anatomy and Physiology of the Penis

"The penis does not obey the order of its master, who tries to erect or shrink it at will. Instead, the penis erects freely while its master is asleep. The penis must be said to have its own mind, by any stretch of the imagination."—Leonardo da Vinci

Historical Aspects

The first description of erectile dysfunction dates from about 2000 BC and was set down on Egyptian papyrus. Two types were described: natural impotence ("the man is incapable of accomplishing the sex act") and supernatural impotence (arising from evil charms and spells). Later, Hippocrates described many cases of male impotence among the rich inhabitants of Scythia and concluded that too much horseback riding was the cause (the poor were not affected because they traveled on foot).

Aristotle stated that three branches of nerves carry spirit and energy to the penis and that erection is produced by an influx of air.[1] His theory was well accepted until 1504, when Leonardo da Vinci noted the presence of a large amount of blood in the erect penises of hanged men, casting doubt on the concept of the air-filled penis. In 1585, Ambroise Pare accurately described the penile anatomy and the concept of erection in his *Ten Books on Surgery* and *Book of Reproduction*. Pare described the penis as being composed of concentric coats of nerves, veins, and arteries, two ligaments (corpora cavernosa), a urinary tract, and four muscles. He wrote, "When the man becomes inflamed with lust and desire, blood rushes into the male member and causes it to become erect."

Much progress has been made since the 16th century in the understanding of erectile anatomy, function, and dysfunction. Many theories have since been advanced to explain the hemodynamic events that occur during erection and detumescence. In the 19th century, venous occlusion was believed to be the main factor in achieving and maintaining erection. Later, investigators stressed the importance of increased arterial blood flow. Controversies about the mechanism of erection continued until the late 1970s and early 1980s, when studies in human volunteers and animal models began to shed light on the anatomic and hemodynamic changes that occur during erection. These studies resolved many of the uncertainties.

In the last decade, intensive research has yielded many important breakthroughs, most notably the identification of nitric oxide (NO) as the chief neurotransmitter for erection. The role of smooth muscle in regulat-

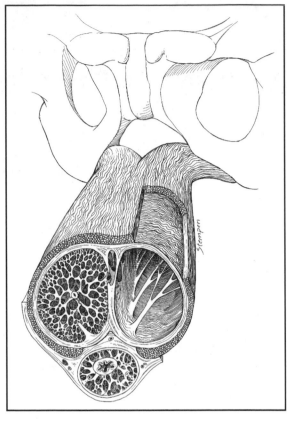

Figure 1-1: Cross-section of the penis showing the intracavernous pillars supporting the erectile tissue and the inner circular and outer longitudinal layers of the tunica albuginea. The longitudinal layer is absent between the corpus cavernosum and the spongiosum. Used with permission from Walsh PC, Retik AB, Vaughan ED Jr, et al, eds: *Campbell's Urology*, 7th ed. Philadelphia, WB Saunders, 1997, chapter 38.

ing arterial and venous flow and the detailed structure and function of the tunica albuginea also have been elucidated. In pathophysiology, the changes to the smooth muscle, endothelium, and fibroelastic framework induced by diabetes, atherosclerosis, and aging also have been identified.

Functional Anatomy of the Penis
Tunica Albuginea

The tunica encloses and protects the erectile tissue. During erection, the tunica allows for controlled expansion while providing rigidity and supporting other components of the penis (Figure 1-1). The tunical covering of the corpora cavernosa is a bilayered structure with multiple sublayers. Inner-layer bundles, oriented circularly, support and contain the cavernous tissue. Intracavernosal pillars acting as struts radiate from this inner layer, augmenting the septum. Together, these structures provide essential support to the erectile tissue. Outer-layer bundles are oriented longitudinally, extending from the glans penis to the proximal crus. The bundles attach to the inferior pubic ramus but are absent between the 5- and 7-o'clock positions. In contrast to the corpora cavernosa, the corpus

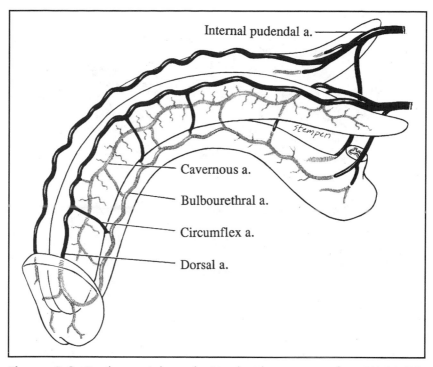

Figure 1-2: Penile arterial supply. Used with permission from Walsh PC, Retik AB, Vaughan ED Jr, et al, eds: *Campbell's Urology*, 7th ed. Philadelphia, WB Saunders, 1997, chapter 38.

spongiosum lacks an outer layer and intracorporeal struts, and the circular inner layer is much thinner, which ensures a relatively low-pressure structure during erection.

The tunica itself is composed of elastic fibers that form an irregular lattice network on which collagen fibers rest. The arteries (the cavernous and collaterals between the dorsal and cavernous) enter the corpus cavernosum surrounded by a cuff of periarterial loose areolar tissue, which protects the arteries from being closed off by the tunica during erection. On the other hand, the emissary veins penetrate the layers of tunica albuginea without a perivascular cuff and are easily 'strangulated' by tunical stretching during erection.

The outer tunical layer largely determines the variability in tunical thickness and strength.[2] Strength and thickness correlate significantly with location. The tunica is thicker and stronger in the periurethral ridge and the dorsum but is thinner between the cavernosum and the spongiosum. This is the weakest area of the tunica. As a result of this vulnerability, most prostheses tend to extrude here.

Corpora Cavernosa, Corpus Spongiosum, and Glans Penis

The corpora cavernosa are composed of two spongy, paired cylinders

7

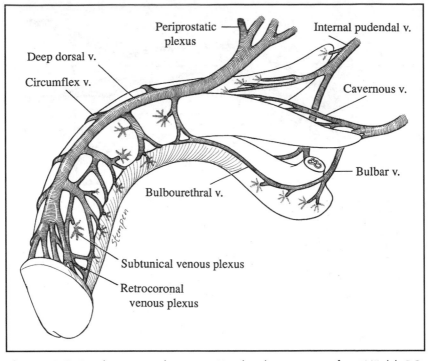

Figure 1-3: Penile venous drainage. Used with permission from Walsh PC, Retik AB, Vaughan ED Jr, et al, eds: *Campbell's Urology*, 7th ed. Philadelphia, WB Saunders, 1997, chapter 38.

in the thick envelope of the tunica albuginea. Their proximal ends, the crura, attach to the undersurface of the puboischial rami as two separate structures. The crura merge under the pubic arch and remain attached up to the glans. The septum between the two corpora cavernosa is fenestrated in men but is complete in some species, such as canines.

The corpora cavernosa are supported by a fibrous skeleton that includes the tunica albuginea, intracavernous pillars, the intracavernous fibrous framework, and the periarterial and perineural fibrous sheath.[3] Within these frameworks are interconnected vascular spaces (sinusoids, or lacunar spaces) lined by endothelial cells. Each corpus cavernosum is a conglomeration of sinusoids, larger in the center and smaller in the periphery. In the flaccid state, the blood-gas levels in the sinusoid are similar to those of venous blood. During erection, the rapid entry of arterial blood to sinusoids changes the intracavernous blood-gas levels to those of arterial blood.

The structures of the corpus spongiosum and glans are similar to those of the corpora cavernosa, except that the sinusoids are larger. Moreover, the tunica is thinner in the spongiosum, composed of a single circular layer that is completely absent in the glans.

Why the os penis disappeared from the human male

In evolutionary history, many vertebrates have featured a piece of bone, the os penis, attached to the corpus cavernosum to enhance its rigidity. When vertebrates started to become bipedal, the os penis became a selective disadvantage because it was easily damaged in combat. Primates, who are partially bipedal, have a vestigial piece of the os penis, smaller in proportion than that of quadrupeds. When primates evolved into human beings, the os penis disappeared. As a result, the flaccid penis of the human became less susceptible to injury in contact sport.

However, with the disappearance of the os penis came a kind of evolutionary compensation. Because of the absence of a rigid bone, the tunica albuginea in humans is much thicker than that of the canine and primate, and it provides a more rigid penis with the same intracavernous pressure. For example, 100 mm Hg of intracavernous pressure in dogs and monkeys yields only partial rigidity. Only with the contraction of the ischiocavernosus muscle, which raises the pressure to several hundred mm Hg, will the penis achieve full rigidity. On the other hand, 100 mm Hg of intracavernous pressure in a human penis produces a very firm organ because of its thicker tunica and larger diameter.

Arterial Supply

The main source of blood to the penis is usually the internal pudendal artery, a branch of the internal iliac artery. However, accessory arteries arising from the external iliac, obturator, vesical, and femoral arteries may occasionally become the dominant or only arterial supply to the corpus cavernosum. The internal pudendal artery becomes the common penile artery after branching off to the perineum. The three main branches of the penile artery are the cavernous, dorsal, and bulbourethral arteries (Figure 1-2).

Entering at the hilum of the penis, where the two crura merge, the cavernous artery is responsible for tumescence of the corpus cavernosum. Along its course, the cavernous artery branches off many helicine arteries, which supply blood to the trabecular erectile tissue and the sinusoids. These helicine arteries are contracted and tortuous in the flaccid state and become dilated and straight during erection. The dorsal artery supplies blood to the skin and subcutaneous tissue and is responsible for engorgement of the glans penis during erection. The bulbourethral artery supplies blood to the bulb and corpus spongiosum. The three branches join distally to form a vascular ring near the glans (Figure 1-2).

Venous Drainage

The venous drainage from the three corpora originates in tiny venules leading from the peripheral sinusoids immediately beneath the tunica albuginea. These venules travel in the trabeculae between the tunica and the peripheral sinusoids to form the sub-

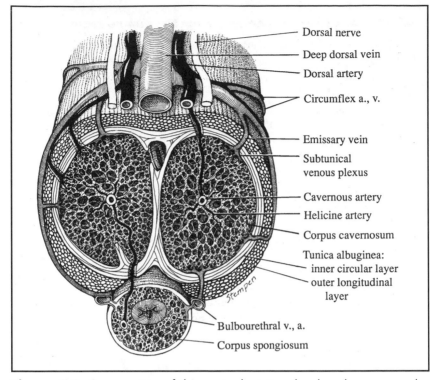

Figure 1-4: Cross-section of the penis depicting the dorsal neurovascular bundle, potential communications between the dorsal, cavernous, and urethral arteries, and the rich anastomosis between the veins draining the corpora cavernosa and those draining the corpus spongiosum. Used with permission from Walsh PC, Retik AB, Vaughan ED Jr, et al, eds: *Campbell's Urology*, 7th ed. Philadelphia, WB Saunders, 1997, chapter 38.

tunicary venular plexus before exiting as the emissary veins (Figures 1-3 and 1-4). Outside the tunica albuginea, the venous drainage occurs as follows:

Skin and subcutaneous tissue. Multiple superficial veins run subcutaneously and unite near the root of the penis to form the superficial dorsal vein, which in turn drains into the saphenous veins. The superficial dorsal vein may also occasionally drain a portion of the corpora cavernosa.

Mid and distal corpora. The emissary veins from the corpus cavernosum and spongiosum drain dorsally to the deep dorsal vein, laterally to the circumflex vein, and ventrally to the periurethral vein. The prominent deep dorsal vein is the main venous drainage of the glans penis and distal two thirds of the corpora cavernosa. Proximally, the deep dorsal vein travels behind the symphysis pubis to join the periprostatic venous plexus.

Infrapubic corpora. Emissary veins that drain the proximal corpora cavernosa join to form cavernous and crural veins. These veins join the peri-

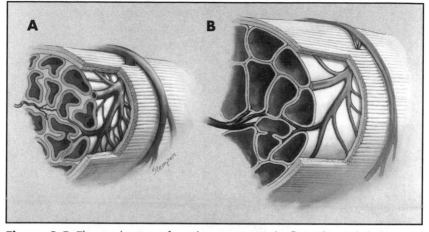

Figure 1-5: The mechanism of penile erection. In the flaccid state (A), the arteries, arterioles, and sinusoids are contracted. The intersinusoidal and subtunicary venular plexuses are wide open, with free flow to the emissary veins. In the erect state (B), the muscles of the sinusoidal wall and the arterioles relax, allowing maximal flow to the compliant sinusoidal spaces. Most venules are compressed between the expanding sinusoids. Even the larger intermediary venules are sandwiched and flattened by distended sinusoids and the noncompliant tunica albuginea. This effectively reduces the venous capacity to a minimum. Used with permission from Walsh PC, Retik AB, Vaughan ED Jr, et al, eds: *Campbell's Urology*, 7th ed. Philadelphia, WB Saunders, 1997, chapter 38.

urethral veins from the urethral bulb to form the internal pudendal vein.

The veins of the three systems communicate variably with one another. Variations among patients in the number, distribution, and termination of the venous systems are common.

Hemodynamics and Mechanism of Erection and Detumescence

Corpora Cavernosa

The penile erectile tissues, specifically the cavernous smooth musculature and the smooth muscles of the arteriolar and arterial walls, are key in the erectile process. In the flaccid state, these smooth muscles are partially contracted by the sympathetic discharge, allowing only a small amount of arterial flow for nutritional purposes. Thus, the flaccid penis is in a moderate state of contraction, as evidenced by further shrinkage in cold weather.

Sexual stimulation triggers release of neurotransmitters and the following events (Figure 1-5): (1) relaxation of the smooth muscles in the arteriolar and arterial walls, resulting in dilation of the arterioles and arteries and increased blood flow; (2) trapping of incoming blood by the expanding sinusoids; (3) compression of the subtunicary venular plexuses between the tunica albuginea and the peripheral trabeculae, reducing the venous outflow; (4) stretching of the tunica to its capacity, thereby strangulating the

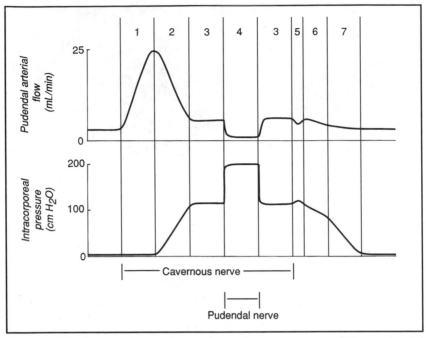

Figure 1-6: During electrostimulation of the cavernous and the pudendal nerves in a canine model, seven phases of penile erection and detumescence are noted: 1, latent; 2, tumescence; 3, full erection; 4, rigid erection; 5, early detumescence; 6, slow detumescence; 7, fast detumescence. Used with permission from Walsh PC, Retik AB, Vaughan ED Jr, et al, eds: *Campbell's Urology,* 7th ed. Philadelphia, WB Saunders, 1997, chapter 38.

emissary veins between the tunical layers and further decreasing venous outflow to a minimum; (5) an increase in intracavernous pressure (maintained around 100 mm Hg), which raises the penis from the dependent position to the erect state (full erection); and (6) a further pressure increase to several hundred mm Hg, with contraction of the ischiocavernosus muscles (rigid erection). The angle of the erect penis is determined by its size and its attachment to the anterior surface of the pubic bone (the suspensory and funiform ligaments). In patients with a long, heavy penis or loose suspensory ligament, the angle usually will not be greater than 90°, even with full rigidity.

Three phases of detumescence have been observed in our animal study. The first phase entails a transient intracorporeal pressure increase, indicating the beginning of smooth muscle contraction against a closed venous system. The second phase involves a slow pressure decrease, suggesting a slow reopening of the venous channels with resumption of the basal level of arterial flow. The third phase involves a fast pressure decrease with fully restored venous outflow capacity.

Why are vascular organs (corpus cavernosum and spongiosum) critical for sexual function?

An interesting speculation is why vascular tissue has gained an advantage over other kinds of tissues for penile erection. Bony or fibrous tissues are out of the question because both would just protrude from the body, and neither can be controlled by nerves. Striated muscle has the dual disadvantages of potential fatigue and purely voluntary (somatic) control. Imagine if a man could erect his penis instantaneously any time he wished. Our work schedules and moral standards would undoubtedly suffer. In addition, a bony support would be needed to enhance penile rigidity. Without it, penile size would have to be quite large to attain the rigidity suitable for the sexual act. Three-legged pants would become the standard dress for men. Even with a bony support, fracture of the os penis would become a common sports injury.

In my opinion, the advantages of using vascular tissue for the penis are several: (1) once blood rushes in and the venous system shuts off, the penis becomes several times larger and can be maintained with little effort so that a man can spend his energy on other activities; (2) with its thick tunica albuginea, the vascular organ can become a rigid pipe that supports the ejaculatory apparatus—the spongiosum and the glans; (3) the vascular corpus spongiosum not only can provide a pressurized chamber for the expulsion of ejaculate, but also can become a large lumen for urination in the flaccid state; and (4) when the blood is out of the system, the penis is smaller and soft, lessening the chances of injury.

Erection thus involves sinusoidal relaxation, arterial dilation, and venous compression.[4] The seven distinct hemodynamic phases of erection and detumescence and the relationship between penile arterial flow and intracavernous pressure are depicted in Figure 1-6.

Corpus Spongiosum and Glans Penis

The hemodynamics of the corpus spongiosum and glans penis are somewhat different from those of the corpora cavernosa. During erection, arterial flow in the corpus spongiosum increases similarly to that in the corpora cavernosa. However, the pressure in the corpus spongiosum and glans is only one third to one half that in the corpora cavernosa because the tunical covering (thin over the corpus spongiosum and virtually absent over the glans) ensures minimal venous occlusion. During full erection, partial compression of the deep dorsal and circumflex veins contributes to tumescence of the glans. The spongiosum and glans function as a large arteriovenous shunt during this phase. In the rigid erection phase, the spongiosum and penile veins are forcibly compressed by the ischiocavernosus and bulbocavernosus

Table 1-1: The Function of Penile Components During Penile Erection

Corpora cavernosa	• Support corpus spongiosum and glans
Tunica albuginea (of corpora cavernosa)	• Protects erectile tissue • Provides rigidity • Participates in veno-occlusive mechanism
Smooth muscle	• Regulates blood flow into and out of the sinusoids
Ischiocavernosus muscle	• Pumps blood distally to speed up erection • Provides additional penile rigidity during rigid erection phase
Bulbocavernosus muscle	• Compresses the bulb and urethra to help expel semen
Corpus spongiosum	• Provides a pressurized narrow chamber to allow expulsion of semen from urethra
Glans	• Acts as a cushion to lessen the impact of the penis on female organs • Provides sensory input to facilitate erection and enhance pleasure • Cone shape facilitates intromission

muscles, which results in further engorgement and increased pressure in the glans and spongiosum.

Function of Various Penile Components

The components in the penis (Table 1-1) serve two main functions: urination and sexual intercourse. The spongy tissues within the corpus cavernosum provide the physical space for trapping and storage of blood during erection. To regulate inflow and outflow, nerve-controlled smooth muscles line the arteries, arterioles, and the trabeculae. If we consider only this process, the penis works just like a sponge, soaking up blood and becoming enlarged during erection but with no rigidity.

The bilayered tunica albuginea works like a soft shell to which the trabeculae attach when the penis is flaccid. During erection, the tunica albuginea and the intracavernous pillars stretch to their maximum length and provide rigidity to the blood-filled corpora cavernosa. With their attachment to the ischial bone, the corpora cavernosa can protrude from the body and become rigid supporting beams for the glans penis and the urethra. The striated ischiocavernosus muscle has no function in the flaccid state but becomes an *erection enhancer*. Its muscle fibers wrap around the base of

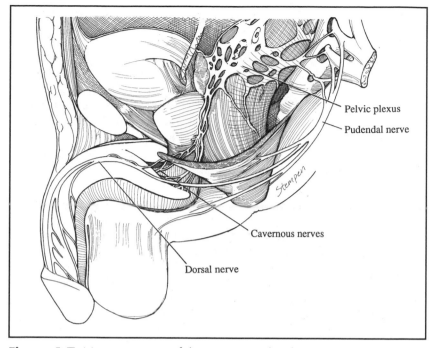

Figure 1-7: Neuroanatomy of the penis. Used with permission from Walsh PC, Retik AB, Vaughan ED Jr, et al, eds: *Campbell's Urology*, 7th ed. Philadelphia, WB Saunders, 1997, chapter 38.

the corpora cavernosa, while its tendons pass into the longitudinal layers of the tunica albuginea. During erection, contraction of this muscle and the bulbocavernosus muscle (resulting from the bulbocavernous reflex triggered by masturbation or sexual act) temporarily shuts off all venous return from the penis and compresses the blood-filled corpora cavernosa and spongiosum. As a result, the glans engorges further, the penile angle increases, the intracavernous pressure jumps to several hundred mm Hg, and the penis becomes fully rigid. With the interaction and cooperation of the brain, nerves, blood, fibroelastic sheath, and smooth and striated muscle, the penis is transformed from

a 'wet noodle' to 'blue steel,' two interesting descriptive terms used by some of my patients.

The corpus spongiosum, with its centrally located urethra, is a capacious elastic tube designed to accommodate passage of several hundred mL of urine within several minutes (up to 50 mL/ sec peak flow rate). The corpus spongiosum can also collapse to seal off its lumen and prevent air or bacteria from traveling upward to the bladder. During erection, the corpus spongiosum engorges to add girth to the penis and provide a pressurized passage for semen ejaculation. If the urethra is not converted to a pressurized and narrowed chamber (similar to the barrel of a rifle), the semen, which only con-

Multiple nerve controls (autonomic and somatic) ensure penile function

Considering the importance of the penis in the propagation of the human species, we should not be surprised at the apparent redundancy of nerve controls in the penis. In the resting state, the flaccid penis is maintained by the action of extrinsic (sympathetic) and intrinsic (endothelial) factors that maintain the muscles in a semicontracted state. Penile erection can be produced by autonomic impulse alone, as in nocturnal penile erection (subconscious) and audiovisual sexual stimulation (conscious). Erection can also be initiated by genital stimulation (somatic sensory impulses), which signals the erection centers in the brain and the spinal cord to send nerve impulses to the penis (parasympathetic and nonadrenergic/noncholinergic impulses) and the ischiocavernosus muscle (somatic motor impulses). This multiple, overlapping control mechanism ensures that a single system failure will not impair penile function.

Autonomic nerve control is essential in the penis. The organ itself is flaccid about 22 hours a day, and the erectile tissues are bathed in a relatively acidic and oxygen-poor environment. If men were granted full voluntary control of their erections, some might decide to stop their erections altogether for several years, while others would be erect 24 hours a day! Both extremes would cause damage and irreversible structural alterations. Autonomic nerve control ensures that a man cannot overuse or underuse his penis. Several episodes of erection every night replenish the penile tissues with nutrients, oxygen, growth factors, and many unknown molecules to ensure a well-serviced organ that is ready for function when needed. However, because of the unpredictable availability of a sexual partner, some voluntary control is necessary so a man can perform when opportunities arise. Therefore, sensory input from genital and audiovisual stimulation enhances and modulates the man's autonomic control.

stitutes 2 to 5 mL, would simply remain in the urethra and later dribble out with urine during urination.

The cone-shaped glans penis also has multiple functions. In urination, the glans works like a control head of a garden hose to help form a stream. The fossa navicularis just inside the glans helps retain one or two drops of urine so the urethra mucosa do not dry up and crack. For sexual function, the cone shape makes intromission easier, and the enlarged head helps prevent semen from escaping from the vagina after ejaculation. Moreover, its spongelike characteristics work as a cushion to absorb the impact of the penis on the cervix.

The bulbocavernosus muscle is a striated muscle wrapped around the bulb of the urethra. After urination, its contraction helps push out the last few drops of urine. During ejaculation, its rhythmic contraction helps propel the semen through the pressurized urethra.

Neuroanatomy and Neurophysiology of Penile Erection

Peripheral Pathways

The innervation of the penis is autonomic (sympathetic and parasympathetic) and somatic (sensory and motor) (Figure 1-7). From neurons in the spinal cord and peripheral ganglia, the sympathetic and parasympathetic nerves merge to form the cavernous nerves, which enter the corpora cavernosa and corpus spongiosum to trigger the neurovascular events during erection and detumescence. The somatic nerves are primarily responsible for penile sensation and contraction of the bulbocavernosus and ischiocavernosus muscles.

Autonomic Pathways

The sympathetic pathway originates from the 11th thoracic to the 2nd lumbar spinal segments and passes through various structures to the pelvic plexus. In men, the T_{11} to T_{12} segments are most often the origin of the sympathetic fibers.

The parasympathetic pathway arises from neurons in the intermediolateral cell columns of the 2nd, 3rd, and 4th sacral spinal cord segments. The preganglionic fibers pass through the pelvic nerves to the pelvic plexus, where they are joined by the sympathetic nerves from the superior hypogastric plexus.

The cavernous nerves are branches of the pelvic plexus that innervate the penis. Because of their location, these nerves are easily damaged during radical excision of the rectum, bladder, and prostate. A clear understanding of the location and course of these nerves is essential to the prevention of iatrogenic erectile dysfunction.[5]

Stimulation of the pelvic plexus and the cavernous nerves induces erection, whereas stimulation of the hypogastric nerve or the sympathetic trunk causes detumescence. This clearly implies that the sacral parasympathetic input is responsible for tumescence, and the thoracolumbar sympathetic pathway is responsible for detumescence. Many men with sacral spinal cord injury retain psychogenic erectile ability, even though reflexogenic erection ability is abolished. These cerebrally elicited erections occur more often in patients with lower motor neuron lesions below T_{12}. No psychogenic erection occurs in patients with lesions above T_9; the efferent sympathetic outflow is thus suggested to be at T_{11} and T_{12}.

It is, therefore, possible that cerebral impulses normally travel through sympathetic pathways (inhibiting norepinephrine release), parasympathetic pathways (releasing NO and acetylcholine), and somatic pathways (releasing acetylcholine), to produce a normal rigid erection. In patients with a sacral cord lesion, the cerebral impulse can still travel the sympathetic pathway to inhibit norepinephrine release, and NO and acetylcholine can still be released by rerouted synapses with postganglionic parasympathetic and somatic neurons.

Somatic Pathways

The somatosensory pathway originates at sensory receptors in the penile skin, glans, urethra, and within the corpus cavernosum. The human glans penis has numerous afferent terminations: free nerve endings and corpuscular receptors. Nerve fibers from the receptors converge to form the bundles of the penile dorsal nerve, which join other nerves to become the pudendal nerve. Stimulation of these sensory receptors sends messages of pain, temperature, and touch to the thalamus and sensory cortex for sensory perception via the dorsal and pudendal nerves, spinal cord, and spinothalamic tract. The dorsal nerve is a mixed nerve with somatic and autonomic components that enable it to regulate erectile and ejaculatory function.

Motor nuclei in the second to fourth sacral spinal segments are the center of somatomotor penile innervation. These nerves travel in the sacral nerves to the pudendal nerve to innervate the ischiocavernosus and bulbocavernosus muscles. Contraction of the ischiocavernosus muscles produces rigid erection. Rhythmic contraction of the bulbocavernosus muscle is necessary for ejaculation.

Supraspinal Pathways

The central anatomic structures involved in the mediation of erection include the prefrontal cortex, hippocampus, amygdala, hypothalamus, midbrain, pons, and medulla. Supraspinal sites that project directly to the spinal cord center for penile erection include the paraventricular nucleus (PVN), the locus ceruleus, nucleus paragigantocellularis, parapyramidal reticular formation, raphae magnus, raphe pallidus, A5-adrenergic cell group, and Barrington's nucleus.

In response to sexual stimulation, these pathways send inhibitory and excitatory signals to the spinal erection center to modulate the sexual response. At the supraspinal level, the pathways involved in the control of penile erection overlap with the pathways involved in pain and cardiovascular control. Neuroendocrine factors may also modulate central nervous system control of penile erection.

The medial preoptic area (MPOA) and the paraventricular nucleus of the hypothalamus have been identified as important integration centers for sexual drive and penile erection.[6] Animal studies have traced labeled neurons from major pelvic ganglia to neurons in the spinal cord, brain stem, and hypothalamus.[7] Efferent pathways from the MPOA enter the medial forebrain bundle and the midbrain tegmental region (near the substantia nigra). Lesions in these regions (eg, Parkinson's disease, cerebrovascular accidents) are often associated with erectile dysfunction. Many neurotransmitters, including dopamine, norepinephrine, serotonin, oxytocin, and vasopressin, have been identified in the MPOA. The dopaminergic and adrenergic receptors have been shown to promote sexual drive, while serotonin receptors inhibit it.[8]

Neurologic input produces three types of erection: psychogenic, reflexogenic, and nocturnal. Psychogenic erection results from audiovisual stimuli or fantasy. Impulses from the brain modulate the spinal erection centers (T_{11}-L_2 and S_2-S_4), which in turn activate the erectile process. Reflexogenic erection is produced by tactile stimuli to the genitals. Sensory impulses reach the spinal erection centers; some ascend to cortical centers and result in sensory perception, while others activate the autonomic nuclei and the cavernous nerves to induce erection. Nocturnal erection occurs mostly during rapid eye movement (REM) sleep. The mechanism of its activation is unknown.

In the past 3 years, researchers have used positron emission tomography (PET) or functional magnetic resonance imaging (fMRI) to study the change of regional cerebral blood flow (rCBF) in men during visual sexual stimulation. These data were compared with rCBF changes while volunteers watched videos of nonsexual activities such as sports and news. These studies began to shed light on the brain processing of visual sexual stimuli and have identified several brain regions with increased or decreased rCBF.[9-11] In PET studies, sexual arousal was mainly associated with activation of bilateral, predominantly right, inferoposterior extrastriate cortices, the right inferolateral prefrontal cortex, and the midbrain. Decreased rCBF was observed in several temporal areas. In fMRI studies, penile turgidity was associated with strong activation of the right subinsular region, including the claustrum, left caudate and putamen, right middle occipital/middle temporal gyri, bilateral cingulate gyrus, and right sensorimotor and premotor regions. Based on these findings, models of brain processing have been proposed on mediating the cognitive, emotional, motivational, and autonomic components of human male sexual arousal.

Neurotransmitters

Peripheral Neurotransmitters for Flaccidity and Detumescence

Adrenergic nerve fibers and receptors have been identified in the cavernous trabeculae and surrounding the cavernous arteries, and norepinephrine has generally been accepted as the principal neurotransmitter in maintaining penile flaccidity at rest and producing detumescence after ejaculation (Figure 1-6).[12] Researchers suggest that sympathetic contraction is mediated by activation of postsynaptic α_1-adrenergic receptors[13] and modulated by presynaptic α_2-adrenergic receptors.[14]

Endothelins, a group of potent vasoconstrictors produced by endothelial cells, also have been suggested as mediators for maintaining penile flaccidity.[15] Other vasoconstrictors, such as thromboxane A2 and prostaglandin $F_{2\alpha}$, have also been proposed.[16]

Erection

Cholinergic nerves have been identified within the human cavernous smooth muscle and surrounding penile arteries, and ultrastructural examination has identified terminals containing cholinergic vesicles in the same area[17] (Figure 1-6). Acetylcholine has been shown to be released with electrical-field stimulation of human erectile tissue. However, intravenous and intracavernous injection of atropine has failed to abolish erection induced in animals by electrical neurostimulation and in men by erotic stimuli.[18] Acetylcholine likely stimulates the release of NO from endothelial cells, thus indirectly contributing to smooth-muscle relaxation and penile erection.[19]

Recent observations strongly suggest that NO released from nonadrenergic/noncholinergic neurons increases the production of cyclic guanine monophosphate (cGMP), which in turn relaxes the cavernous smooth muscle.[20,21] NO-mediated responses are progressively inhibited as a function of decreasing oxygen tension; reverting to normal oxygen tension restores endothelium-dependent and

Table 1-2: Isoforms of Nitric Oxide Synthase (NOS)

Name	Expression	Chromosome	Function
NOS-1 (neuronal)	Constitutive	12	Signal transduction
NOS-2 (inducible)	Induced	17	Antimicrobial Antiparasitic Antineoplastic
NOS-3 (endothelial)	Constitutive	7	Signal transduction

neurogenic relaxation.[22] NO or a NO-like substance seems to be the most likely principal neurotransmitter causing penile erection.

NO is a product of molecular oxygen and L-arginine catalyzed by nitric oxide synthase (NOS) distributed in the vascular endothelium, nerve terminal, and smooth muscle. There are at least three distinct forms of NOS: neuronal, endothelial, and inducible[23] (Table 1-2). In neurons and endothelium, NOS is constitutive and is activated by calcium, which binds calmodulin as an enzyme cofactor. Previous studies have shown that cGMP induces the relaxation of numerous smooth-muscle preparations, including vascular, airway, and intestinal smooth muscle. The mechanisms by which intracellular cGMP promotes smooth-muscle relaxation are still unclear. Possible mechanisms are: (1) activation of cGMP-specific protein kinase resulting in the phosphorylation and inactivation of myosin light-chain kinase and smooth-muscle relaxation; (2) pumping of Ca^{2+} into sarcoplasmic reticulum involving L-type Ca^{2+} channels; (3) activation of cGMP-dependent phosphokinase,

which phosphorylates IP_3 receptors and, therefore, inhibits smooth-muscle contraction; and (4) alteration of potassium channels, resulting in hyperpolarization. Many studies suggest that cGMP is a more potent relaxant of smooth muscle than is cyclic adenosine monophosphate (cAMP).

Other investigators believe that vasoactive intestinal polypeptide (VIP) may be a neurotransmitter responsible for erection. Interestingly, VIP-induced relaxation is reportedly inhibited by the NO synthesis blocker N-ω-nitro-L-arginine. This has led some to suggest that NO production is involved in VIP-stimulated smooth-muscle relaxation. Other potential candidates include calcitonin gene-related peptide (CGRP),[24] peptide histidine methionine,[25] pituitary adenylate cyclase-activating polypeptide,[26] and prostaglandins.[27]

Neuromodulation

Because of the multiple neurotransmitters and endothelial factors involved at the neuromuscular junction, the release of one factor may alter the action of the others on smooth muscle. For example, acetylcholine and VIP seem to be localized in parasympathetic neurons. They may act synergistically to induce erection through inhibition of α-1 activity by acetylcholine and release of NO by VIP.[28] Another example is endothelin-1 (ET-1), which potentiates the action of norepinephrine. NO and ET-1 seem to have a reciprocal relationship in that when the NO level is reduced by a NOS blocker, the vasoconstrictive action of endothelin is up-regulated.[29,30]

Intercellular Communication

Because of the sparse innervation of the cavernous smooth muscles, cells must communicate to mediate synchronized relaxation and contraction. Several studies have demonstrated the presence of gap junctions in the membranes of adjacent muscle cells. These intercellular channels allow for the exchange of ions such as calcium, potassium, and second-messenger molecules.[31] Cell-to-cell communication through these gap junctions most likely explains the synchronized responses that occur during erection and detumescence.

Central Neurotransmitters

A variety of neurotransmitters, including dopamine, norepinephrine, and serotonin, have been identified in the MPOA. Researchers suggest that dopaminergic and adrenergic receptors may promote sexual drive and penile erection and that serotonin receptors inhibit them.

Dopamine. Clinical observations suggest that dopaminergic stimulation increases libido and produces erection. In men, apomorphine, which stimulates D_1 and D_2 receptors, induces penile erection that is unaccompanied by sexual arousal.

Serotonin. Studies indicate that serotonin (5-hydroxytryptamine [5-HT]) pathways inhibit copulation but that 5-HT may have facilitatory and inhibitory effects on sexual function, depending on the receptor subtypes, their location, and species. Some researchers have summarized the results of administration of selective agonists and antagonists as follows: 5-HT-1A receptor agonists inhibit erectile activity but facilitate ejaculation; stimulation of 5-HT-1C receptors causes erection; and 5-HT-2 agonists inhibit erection but facilitate seminal emission and ejaculation. Steers and de Groat have shown increased firing of the cavernous nerve and erection when *m*-chlorophenyl-piperazine (MCPP), a 5-HT-1C/1D receptor agonist, is given to rats.[32] This may partially explain the occasional reports of priapism after the administration of trazodone (Desyrel®), whose metabolites include MCPP.

Noradrenaline. Activation of α_2-adrenoceptors in the MPOA is associated with a decrease in sexual behavior in rats, and administration of clonidine (Catapres®), an α_2-adrenergic agonist, produces impotence and decreased libido in hypertensive patients. Yohimbine (Yocon®, Yohimex™, Aprodyne®, Yovital™), an α_2-receptor antagonist, has been shown to increase sexual activity in castrated rats. However, in impotent men, the clinical effect is only marginal.

Prolactin. Increased levels of prolactin suppress sexual function in men and laboratory animals. In rats, high levels of prolactin decrease the genital reflex and disturb copulatory be-

Table 1-3: Erection-Inducing Agents

Name	Action
Intracavernous and Intraurethral Agents	
Prostaglandins E_1 and E_2	Increase cAMP (receptor-mediated)
Peptides • vasoactive intestinal polypeptide • calcitonin gene-related peptide	Increase cAMP (receptor-mediated)
Alkaloids • papaverine • forskolin	Inhibits phosphodiesterase Increases cAMP (direct action on adenylate cyclase)
α-Adrenergic blockers • phentolamine • moxisylyte	α_1-Adrenoceptor blockers
Nitric oxide donors • nitroprusside	Increase cGMP
Calcium channel blockers	Decrease intracellular calcium
Potassium channel openers	Hyperpolarization
Oral, Sublingual, and Topical Agents	
α-Adrenergic blockers • phentolamine • yohimbine	α_1-Adrenoceptor blocker α_2-Adrenoceptor blocker
Dopaminergic agents • apomorphine	Stimulate dopaminergic receptors
Phosphodiesterase inhibitors • sildenafil	Inhibits type 5 phosphodiesterase
Antidepressants • trazodone	α_1-Adrenoceptor blockers Inhibits serotonin reuptake in brain
Hematologic agents • pentoxifylline	Decrease viscosity of blood
Nitric oxide donors • nitroglycerine gel	Increase cGMP

cAMP = cyclic adenosine monophosphate, cGMP = cyclic guanine monophosphate havior. Researchers suggest that pro-lactin inhibits dopaminergic activity in the MPOA.

Opioids. Endogenous opioids affect sexual function: injection of small amounts of morphine into the MPOA facilitates sexual behavior in rats. Larger doses, however, inhibit penile erection and yawning induced by oxytocin or apomorphine. Researchers suggest that endogenous opioids may inhibit central oxytocinergic transmission.

Oxytocin. Oxytocin is released into the circulation during sexual activity in humans and animals. It produces yawning and penile erection when injected into the paraventricular area in rats. Because neurons in the paraventricular area have been shown to contain NOS, and NOS inhibitors prevent apomorphine- and oxytocin-induced erection, researchers suggest that oxytocin acts on neurons whose activity depends on certain levels of NO.

Other neurotransmitters that play a role are glutamate, substance P, and neuropeptide Y, as well as other neurohormones and modulators such as androgens and pheromones.

Pharmacology of Penile Erection

Because smooth-muscle relaxation is a prerequisite for erection, intracavernous injection of vasoactive drugs can induce erection (muscle relaxants) or detumescence (α-adrenergic agonists). The mechanism of smooth-muscle relaxation in response to various vasodilators is complex and not completely understood, especially when a combination of drugs such as papaverine, phentolamine (Regitine®), and prostaglandin E_1 is used. Table 1-3 summarizes the drugs used

clinically and preclinically for inducing penile erection.

Perspectives

The next step in penile physiology research is to better understand ultrastructural and molecular mechanisms, as well as the functional and structural relationships involved in penile erection and erectile dysfunction. Advances in molecular biology techniques will then allow researchers to identify steps suitable for therapeutic intervention using recombinant growth factors, antibodies, and receptor agonists or antagonists. In addition, specific genes can be transfected to inhibit fibrosis, improve NO production, or enhance smooth-muscle relaxation.

References

1.   Brenot PH: Male impotence—a historical perspective. *L'Esprit du Temps*, France, 1994.

2.   Hsu GL, Brock G, Martinez-Pineiro L, et al: The three-dimensional structure of the human tunica albuginea: anatomical and ultrastructural levels. *Int J Impot Res* 1992;4:117-129.

3.   Goldstein AM, Padma-Nathan H: The microarchitecture of the intracavernosal smooth muscle and the cavernosal fibrous skeleton. *J Urol* 1990;144:1144-1146.

4.   Lue TF, Takamura T, Schmidt RA, et al: Hemodynamics of erection in the monkey. *J Urol* 1983;130:1237-1241.

5.   Walsh PC, Brendler CB, Chang T, et al: Preservation of sexual function in men during radical pelvic surgery. *Md Med J* 1990;39:389-393.

6.   Sachs BD, Meisel RL: The physiology of male sexual behavior. In: Knobil E, Neill JD, Ewing LL, et al, eds. *The Physiology of Reproduction*. New York, Raven Press, 1988, pp 1393-1423.

7. Marson L, Platt KB, McKenna KE: Central nervous system innervation of the penis as revealed by the transneuronal transport of pseudorabies virus. *Neuroscience* 1993;55:263-280.

8. Foreman MM, Wernicke JF: Approaches for the development of oral drug therapies for erectile dysfunction. *Semin Urol* 1990;8:107-112.

9. Redoute J, Stoleru S, Gregoire MC, et al: Brain processing of visual sexual stimuli in human males. *Hum Brain Mapp* 2000;11:162-177.

10. Bocher M, Chisin R, Parag Y, et al: Cerebral activation associated with sexual arousal in response to a pornographic clip: A 15O-H_2O PET study in heterosexual men. *Neuroimage* 2001;14(1 Pt 1):105-117.

11. Arnow BA, Desmond JE, Banner LL, et al: Brain activation and sexual arousal in healthy, heterosexual males. Presented at the annual meeting of the American Urological Association, 2001.

12. Hedlund H, Andersson KE: Comparison of the responses to drugs acting on adrenoreceptors and muscarinic receptors in human isolated corpus cavernosum and cavernous artery. *J Auton Pharmacol* 1985;5:81-88.

13. Christ GJ, Maayani S, Valcic M, et al: Pharmacologic studies of human erectile tissue: characteristics of spontaneous contractions and alterations in alpha-adrenoceptor responsiveness with age and disease in isolated tissues. *Br J Pharmacol* 1990;101:375-381.

14. Saenz de Tejada I, Kim N, Lagan I, et al: Regulation of adrenergic activity in penile corpus cavernosum. *J Urol* 1989; 142:1117-1121.

15. Holmquist F, Andersson KE, Hedlund H: Actions of endothelin on isolated corpus cavernosum from rabbit and man. *Acta Physiol Scand* 1990;139:113-122.

16. Hedlund H, Andersson KE, Fovaeus M, et al: Characterization of contraction-mediating prostanoid receptors in human penile erectile tissues. *J Urol* 1989; 141:182-186.

17. Steers WD, McConnell J, Benson GS: Anatomical localization and some pharmacological effects of vasoactive intestinal polypeptide in human and monkey corpus cavernosum. *J Urol* 1984; 132:1048-1053.

18. Wagner G, Uhrenholdt A: Blood flow measurement by the clearance method in the human corpus cavernosum in the flaccid and erect states. In: Zorgniotti AW, Ross G, eds. *Vasculogenic Impotence.* Proceedings of the First International Conference on Corpus Cavernosum Revascularization. Springfield, IL, Charles C. Thomas, 1980, pp 41-46.

19. Saenz de Tejada I, Goldstein I, Azadzoi K, et al: Impaired neurogenic and endothelium-mediated relaxation of penile smooth muscle from diabetic men with impotence. *N Engl J Med* 1989;320: 1025-1030.

20. Ignarro LJ, Bush PA, Buga GM, et al: Nitric oxide and cyclic GMP formation upon electrical field stimulation cause relaxation of corpus cavernosum smooth muscle. *Biochem Biophys Res Commun* 1990;170:843-850.

21. Burnett AL, Lowenstein CJ, Bredt DS, et al: Nitric oxide: a physiologic mediator of penile erection. *Science* 1992; 257:401-403.

22. Kim N, Vardi Y, Padma-Nathan H, et al: Oxygen tension regulates the nitric oxide pathway. Physiological role in penile erection. *J Clin Invest* 1993;91: 437-442.

23. Lowenstein CJ, Snyder SH: Nitric oxide, a novel biologic messenger. *Cell* 1992;70:705-707.

24. Stief CG, Benard F, Bosch RJ, et al: A possible role for calcitonin-gene-related peptide in the regulation of the smooth muscle tone of the bladder and penis. *J Urol* 1990;143:392-397.

25. Kirkeby HJ, Fahrenkrug J, Holmquist F, et al: Vasoactive intestinal polypeptide (VIP) and peptide histidine methionine (PHM) in human penile cor-

pus cavernosum tissue and circumflex veins: localization and in vitro effects. *Eur J Clin Invest* 1992;22:24-30.

26. Hedlund P, Alm P, Hedlund H, et al: Localization and effects of pituitary adenylate cyclase-activating polypeptide (PACAP) in human penile erectile tissue. *Acta Physiol Scand* 1994;150:103-104.

27. Adaikan PG, Ratnam SS: Pharmacology of penile erection in humans. *Cardiovasc Intervent Radiol* 1988;11:191-194.

28. Aoki H, Matsuzaka J, Yeh KH, et al: Involvement of vasoactive intestinal peptide (VIP) as a humoral mediator of penile erectile function in the dog. *J Androl* 1994;15:174-182.

29. Christ GJ, Richards S, Winkler A: Integrative erectile biology: the role of signal transduction and cell-to-cell communication in coordinating corporal smooth muscle tone and penile erction. *Int J Impot Res* 1997;9:69-84.

30. Adams MA, Banting JD, Maurice DH, et al: Vascular control mechanisms in penile erection: phylogeny and the inevitability of multiple and overlapping systems. *Int J Impot Res* 1997;9:85-91.

31. Christ GJ, Moreno AP, Melman A, et al: Gap junction-mediated intercellular diffusion of Ca^{2+} in cultured human corporal smooth muscle cells. *Am J Physiol* 1992;263:C373-C383.

32. Steers WD, de Groat WC: Effects of m-chlorophenylpiperazine on penile and bladder function in rats. *Am J Physiol* 1989;257:R1441-R1449.

Chapter 2

Pathophysiology of Impotence

"Many cases of male impotence are found among the inhabitants of Scythia. In my opinion this impotence arises from the following cause: too much horse-riding is done by the Scythians."—
Hippocrates (Airs, Waters, Places, V, 2, 22)

Epidemiology

An estimated 10 million to 30 million men suffer from impotence in the United States.[1] The increasing incidence of impotence with age was reported by Kinsey et al in 1948: only 1 in 50 men was affected at age 40, but 1 in 4 was affected by age 65.[2] In 1990, Diokno et al reported that 35% of married men aged 60 years and older suffered from erectile impotence.[3]

A more recent report from the Massachusetts Male Aging Study (MMAS) showed a combined prevalence of minimal, moderate, and complete impotence in 52% of noninstitutionalized men aged 40 to 70 years.[4] The prevalence of complete impotence tripled from 5% to 15% between ages 40 and 70. Subject age was the variable most strongly associated with impotence. After adjustment for age, a higher probability of impotence directly correlated with heart disease, hypertension, diabetes, associated medications, and an index of anger and depression; impotence was inversely correlated with serum dehydroepiandrosterone, high-density lipoprotein (HDL), and an index of dominant personality. Cigarette smoking also was associated with a greater probability of complete impotence in men with heart disease and hypertension.[4]

The epidemiologic studies reconfirm that these vascular risk factors contribute to 'premature' aging of many organs, including the heart and the penis. The high association between myocardial insufficiency and impotence is not surprising because the common penile artery is about the same size as the coronary artery. However, although the effects of a diseased coronary artery on the myocardium have long been recognized, the effects of a stenotic penile artery on the penile erectile tissue are still poorly understood. The stenotic changes in the coronary and penile arteries represent early and reversible stages of the disease process; the changes in myocardium and erectile tissue can be considered *late end-organ disease* and, if severe, are irreparable by current treatment.

Other interesting findings from the MMAS include (1) poor correlation between testosterone levels and impotence, and (2) the insignificance of psychological factors in contributing to impotence in the age group studied. These findings raise an important question: should psychological and hormonal evaluations continue to be performed on every patient, or

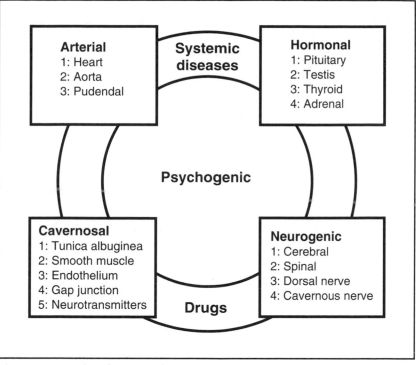

Figure 2-1: Classification of causes of impotence. Used with permission. Carrier et al: *Urology* 1993;42:468-481.

should they be performed only if the history suggests a psychogenic or hormonal cause?

Classification

Many classifications have been proposed for erectile dysfunction. Some are based on the cause (eg, diabetic, iatrogenic, traumatic) and some on the neurovascular mechanism of the erectile process (eg, failure to initiate [neurogenic], failure to fill [arterial], failure to store [venous]). The following classification integrates the various causes of impotence with the modern understanding of erectile physiology and functional anatomy (Figure 2-1).

Psychogenic

Previously, 90% of impotent men were believed to suffer from psychogenic impotence.[5] This belief has given way to the realization that most men with erectile dysfunction have a mixed etiology and that very few suffer from 'pure' psychogenic or organic causes.

Three possible mechanisms may be involved in psychogenic dysfunction: (1) overinhibition of the erection centers by the brain as an exaggeration of the normal suprasacral inhibition, (2) excessive sympathetic outflow or elevated peripheral catecholamine levels, and (3) inadequate release of erectile neurotrans-

Table 2-1: ISIR Classification of Psychogenic Erectile Dysfunction

Generalized Type

- Generalized unresponsiveness
  - primary lack of sexual arousability
  - aging-related decline in sexual arousability

- Generalized inhibition
  - chronic disorder of sexual intimacy

Situational Type

- Partner related
  - lack of arousability in specific relationship
  - lack of arousability caused by sexual object preference
  - high central inhibition caused by partner conflict or threat

- Performance related
  - associated with other sexual dysfunction(s) (eg, rapid ejaculation)
  - situational performance anxiety (eg, fear of failure)

- Psychological distress or adjustment related
  - associated with negative mood state (eg, depression) or major life stress (eg, death of partner)

ISIR = International Society of Impotence Research

---

mitters. Higher levels of serum norepinephrine have been reported in patients with psychogenic erectile impotence than in normal controls or patients with vasculogenic erectile dysfunction.

A subclassification of psychogenic ED has been adopted by the International Society of Impotence Research (Table 2-1):

- Type 1: anxiety, fear of failure (eg, widower's syndrome, sexual phobia, performance anxiety)
- Type 2: depression (including drug- or disease-induced depression)
- Type 3: marital conflict, strained relationship
- Type 4: ignorance and misinformation (eg, about normal anatomy, sexual function, aging), religious scruples
- Type 5: obsessive-compulsive personality (eg, sexual deviation, psychotic disorders)

This subclassification will certainly be modified and improved when the mechanism of various subtypes of psychogenic impotence is better explored and understood.

Neurogenic

Because erection is a neurovascular event, any disease or dysfunction affecting the brain, spinal cord, cavernous and pudendal nerves, or recep-

Table 2-2: Level of Neural Lesion and Its Effect on Erectile Function

Level of the Lesion	Functional Changes
Hypothalamus	Loss of erection, libido, and orgasm
Complete upper spinal cord	Phase 1: prolonged reflex erection may occur for several days (neurogenic priapism) Phase 2: no erection or ejaculation for weeks or months Phase 3: return of reflex erection but not reflex ejaculation
Cord lesion (above T_{12}); sympathetic nerves involved	Autonomic dysreflexia Psychogenic erection absent
Cord lesion (below T_{12}); sympathetic nerves preserved	Psychogenic erection present
Sacral cord (S_2-S_4)	Loss of genital sensation Loss of reflex erection and ejaculation Psychogenic erection may occur
Conus medullaris	Mixed pattern
Cavernous nerves	Loss of psychogenic, reflexogenic, and nocturnal erections Intact genital sensation Normal ejaculation and orgasm
Dorsal nerve of penis	Inability to sustain erection Loss of genital sensation No orgasm or ejaculation May have normal nocturnal erections

Modified with permission from Melman A, Rehman J: Pathophysiology of erectile dysfunction. In: Vaughan ED Jr, Perlmutter AP, eds. *Atlas of Clinical Urology, Vol. 1, Impotence and Infertility*. Philadelphia, Current Medicine, 1999, pp 1.1-1.16.

tors in the terminal arterioles and cavernous smooth muscles can cause erectile dysfunction (Table 2-2).

The medial preoptic area (MPOA) and the paraventricular nucleus are regarded as important integration centers for sexual drive and penile erection in animal studies. Pathologic processes in these regions, such as Parkinson's disease and stroke, are often associated with erectile dysfunction. Parkinsonism may be caused by

Neurogenic impotence may be the most prevalent

In my opinion, neurogenic deficiency may be the most common type of impotence in older men, based on the following observations: (1) animal studies have showed a clear decrease in nitric oxide synthase-containing neurons in the pelvic ganglia and penis of aged rats; and (2) up to 90% of impotent patients can achieve a sustained good erection after intracavernous injection of a trimix solution (a mixture of papaverine, phentolamine, and alprostadil), suggesting that the deficiency is most likely attributable to inadequate neurotransmitter release.

the imbalance of dopaminergic pathways. Other lesions in the brain associated with erectile dysfunction are tumors, Alzheimer's disease lesions, and trauma.

In patients with spinal cord injury, the degree of erectile function that persists depends largely on the nature, location, and extent of the lesion. Reflexogenic erection is preserved in 95% of patients with complete upper cord lesions, whereas only about 25% of those with complete lower cord lesions can achieve an erection.[6] Sacral parasympathetic neurons seem important in the preservation of reflexogenic erection. On the other hand, the thoracolumbar pathway may compensate for loss of the sacral center through synaptic connections.[7] Other disorders at the spinal level (eg, spina bifida, disk herniation, syringomyelia, tumor, multiple sclerosis) may affect the afferent or the efferent neural pathway, resulting in impotence.

Because of the close relationship between the cavernous nerves and the pelvic organs, surgery on these organs frequently causes impotence. The incidence of iatrogenic impotence from various procedures has been reported: radical prostatectomy, 43% to 100%[8,9]; perineal prostatectomy, 29%[8]; abdominal perineal resection, 15% to 100%[10]; and external sphincterotomy at the 3- and 9-o'clock positions, 2% to 49%. An improved understanding of the neuroanatomy of the pelvic and cavernous nerves[11] has resulted in modified surgery for cancer of the rectum, bladder, and prostate, resulting in a lower incidence of iatrogenic impotence. For example, the introduction of nerve-sparing radical prostatectomy has reduced the incidence of impotence from nearly 100% to between 30% and 50%.[12] In cases of pelvic fracture, erectile dysfunction can result from cavernous nerve injury, vascular insufficiency, or both (Table 2-3).

Alcoholism, vitamin deficiency, and diabetes may affect the cavernous or dorsal nerve terminals and may result in deficiency of neurotransmitters. In patients with diabetes, impairment of neurogenic and endothelium-dependent relaxation results in inadequate nitric oxide (NO) release.[13] Recently, nicotinamide adenine dinucleotide phosphate (NADP) diaphorase staining of the nonadrenergic, noncholinergic nerve fibers in penile biopsy specimens has been

Table 2-3: Neurogenic Causes and Prevalence of Impotence

Central Nervous System Disorders

- Parkinson's disease: 60%

- Multiple sclerosis: 70%

- Cerebrovascular accident: 30%

- Others: temporal lobe epilepsy, head trauma, tumor: unknown

- Spinal cord: tumor, trauma, degenerative diseases
  - suprasacral lesions: 5%-10%
  - sacral lesions: 60%-80%

Peripheral Neuropathy

- Diabetes: may involve somatic and autonomic nerves (35%-70%)

- Alcoholism: autonomic neuropathy: unknown

- Aging: loss of pressure, touch, and vibratory sensation: unknown

- Chronic renal failure: autonomic neuropathy: unknown

- Others: scleroderma; lupus; hypothyroidism; vitamin B_1, B_2, and B_6 deficiencies; amyloidosis; industrial toxins; AIDS: unknown

Postsurgical

- Aortoiliac vascular bypass: 30%

- Abdominoperineal resection: 20%-60%

- Transurethral resection of prostate: 4%

- Radical prostatectomy: 40%-70%

Posttraumatic

- Pelvic fracture: 50%

- Perineal injury, bicycle injury: unknown

Modified with permission from Melman A, Rehman J: Pathophysiology of erectile dysfunction. In: Vaughan ED Jr, Perlmutter AP, eds. *Atlas of Clinical Urology, Vol. 1, Impotence and Infertility*. Philadelphia, Current Medicine, 1999, pp 1.1-1.16.

proposed as an indicator of neurologic status.[14]

In impotent patients with no clinically apparent neurologic disease, Bemelmans et al found that 47% had at least one abnormal neurophysiologic measurement and that an abnormality was found more often in

The effects of testosterone

Many of my patients have been given testosterone preparations by their family physicians or urologists before coming to see me. In the MMAS, testosterone had virtually no association with impotence. However, millions of dollars are spent every year because of the false belief that testosterone boosts sexual drive and, therefore, improves potency. Because of the high incidence of prostate cancer in older men, the indiscriminate prescription of testosterone may speed the growth of many microscopic prostate cancers and pose a real threat to a patient's well-being. Before giving testosterone to any man older than 45 years, a detailed prostate examination (including prostate-specific antigen test and, if necessary, prostate ultrasound and biopsy) is strongly recommended.

older patients.[15] A decrease in penile tactile sensitivity with increasing age was also reported by Rowland et al.[16] Sensory input from the genitalia is essential in achieving and maintaining reflexogenic erection, and the input becomes even more important when older men gradually lose psychogenic erection. Therefore, sensory evaluation should be integral to the evaluation for erectile dysfunction in all patients with or without an apparent neurologic disorder.

Endocrinologic

Androgens affect the growth and development of the male reproductive tract and secondary sex characteristics; their effects on libido and sexual behavior are well established. Androgen receptors have been found in the sacral parasympathetic cord and in the hypothalamus and limbic system, suggesting a possible role for central control and influence of erection. Hypogonadal men have decreased nocturnal penile erectile activity that responds to androgen replacement.[17] Others have shown that erection in response to visual sexual stimulation is not affected by androgen withdrawal in hypogonadal men, suggesting that androgens enhance but are not essential for erection.[18] In addition, exogenous testosterone therapy in impotent men with borderline low testosterone levels reportedly has little effect on potency.[19]

Any dysfunction of the hypothalamic-pituitary axis can result in hypogonadism. Hypogonadotropic hypogonadism can be congenital or caused by a tumor or injury; hypergonadotropic hypogonadism may result from a testicular tumor, injury, surgery, or mumps orchitis (Table 2-4).

Hyperprolactinemia, whether from a pituitary adenoma or drugs, results in reproductive and sexual dysfunction (Table 2-5). Symptoms may include loss of libido, erectile dysfunction, galactorrhea, gynecomastia, and infertility. Hyperprolactinemia is associated with low circulating levels of testosterone, which appear to be secondary to inhibition of gonadotropin-releasing hormone secretion by the elevated prolactin.[20]

Erectile dysfunction also may be associated with hyperthyroidism and

Table 2-4: Causes of Hypogonadism (Low Serum Testosterone)

Hypogonadotropic Hypogonadism (low FSH and LH)
Hypothalamic disorders (GnRH deficiency)
- Hypothalamic lesions (tumors, encephalitis, granulomas, craniopharyngioma)
- Isolated GnRH deficiency (idiopathic; associated with Kallmann's syndrome)
- Hyperprolactinemia
- Hemochromatosis
- Aging

Pituitary disorders (gonadotropin deficiency)
- Isolated LH deficiency
- Tumors, infarction
- Empty sella syndrome
- Hemochromatosis

Hypergonadotropic Hypogonadism (high FSH and LH)
Testicular disorders (primary gonadal failure)
- Undescended testes
- Acquired: bilateral torsion of testes, orchitis, tumor, injury, or surgery
- Seminiferous tubule dysgenesis (Klinefelter's syndrome)
- Noonan's (Ullrich-Turner) syndrome
- Hemochromatosis
- Androgen-resistant states and enzyme defects
- Testicular feminization (absence of androgen receptors)
- Incomplete androgen insensitivity (Reifenstein's syndrome)
- 5-α reductase deficiency (pseudovaginal perineal scrotal hypospadias/familial incomplete male) pseudohermaphroditism

Modified with permission from Melman A, Rehman J: Pathophysiology of erectile dysfunction. In: *Atlas of Clinical Urology, Vol. 1, Impotence and Infertility.* Philadelphia, Current Medicine, 1999, pp 1.1-1.16.

FSH = follicle-stimulating hormone, GnRH = gonadotropin-releasing hormone, LH = luteinizing hormone

Table 2-5: Hyperprolactinemia

Hypothalamic Causes

- Tumors
- Granulomas (sarcoidosis, histiocytosis X, tuberculoma)

Pituitary Causes

- Functioning tumors: microadenoma or macroadenoma
- Nonfunctioning tumors
- Stalk section: surgical trauma, meningioma

Pharmaceutical Causes

- Drugs that decrease synthesis of or inhibit release of dopamine; these drugs release lactotrophs from their hypothalamic inhibition and result in overproduction of prolactin
- Drugs that deplete central dopamine stores: methyldopa, reserpine
- Dopamine receptor-blocking agents: chlorpromazine, butyrophenones (haloperidol), benzamides (metoclopramide, sulpiride, domperidone)
- Drugs that block the effect of endogenous dopamine: metoclopramide, amoxapine, verapamil, cocaine, cimetidine, opioids

Miscellaneous Disorders

- Primary hypothyroidism
- Diabetes
- Chronic renal failure
- Liver cirrhosis

Modified with permission from Melman A, Rehman J: Pathophysiology of erectile dysfunction. In: Vaughan ED Jr, Perlmutter AP, eds. *Atlas of Clinical Urology, Vol. 1, Impotence and Infertility*. Philadelphia, Current Medicine, 1999, pp 1.1-1.16.

hypothyroidism. Hyperthyroidism is commonly associated with diminished libido, which may be caused by increased circulating estrogen levels. Hyperthyroidism is less often associated with erectile dysfunction. In hypothyroidism, low testosterone secretion and elevated prolactin levels contribute to erectile dysfunction.

Diabetes mellitus, the most common endocrinologic disorder, causes erectile dysfunction through its vascular, neurologic, endothelial, muscular, and psychogenic complications, rather than hormone deficiency per se. Changes in the cavernous arteries[21] and cavernous erectile tissue[13] have been reported.

Arteriogenic

Atherosclerotic or traumatic arterial occlusive disease of the hypogastric-cavernous-helicine arterial tree can decrease the perfusion pressure and blood flow to the sinusoid spaces, thus increasing the time to full erection and decreasing the rigidity of the erect penis.

Michal and Ruzbarsky found that the incidence and age at onset of coronary disease and erectile dysfunction are parallel.[21] In most patients with arteriogenic erectile dysfunction, the impaired penile perfusion is a component of the generalized atherosclerotic process. Common risk factors associated with arterial insufficiency include hypertension, hyperlipidemia, low HDL, cigarette smoking, diabetes mellitus, blunt perineal or pelvic trauma, and pelvic irradiation.[22,23] On arteriography, bilateral diffuse disease of the internal pudendal, common penile, and cavernous arteries has been found in impotent patients with atherosclerosis. Focal stenosis of the common penile or cavernous artery is most common in young patients who have sustained blunt pelvic or perineal trauma or have repeated minor trauma from long-distance biking.[23] In one report, diabetic men and older men had a high incidence of fibrotic lesions of the cavernous artery, with intimal proliferation, calcification, and luminal stenosis.[21]

Hyperlipidemia is a well-known risk factor for arteriosclerosis. It enhances the deposition of lipid in the vascular wall, causing atherosclerosis and eventual occlusion. Nicotine may adversely affect erectile function by decreasing arterial flow to the penis and blocking corporeal smooth-muscle relaxation, thus preventing normal venous occlusion.[24,25] Hypertension is another well-recognized risk factor for arteriosclerosis; a prevalence of about 45% has been noted in one series of impotent men.[25] However, in hypertension, the increased blood pressure itself does not impair erectile function; rather, the associated arterial stenotic lesions are believed to be the cause.[26]

Thanks to public education, exercise, smoking cessation, diet modification, and medications, the incidence of myocardial infarction has declined in recent years. In early penile arterial disease, the alterations in the artery and erectile tissue are reversible, and changes in lifestyle and eating habits may correct the problem. However, in most cases, the disease process already involves the cavernous smooth muscles (end-organ failure), and reversal of the process becomes more difficult.

Cavernosal (Venogenic)

Failure of adequate venous occlusion has been proposed as one of the most common causes of vasculogenic impotence. Veno-occlusive dysfunction may result from several pathophysiologic processes (Table 2-6).

Fibroelastic component. Loss of compliance of the penile sinusoids may result from aging and its increased deposition of collagen[27] associated with hypercholesterolemia. Altered collagen synthesis also may hinder compliance. Alterations in the fibroelastic structures can also occur after penile trauma or priapism.

Smooth muscle. Wespes et al demonstrated a decrease in the smooth-muscle fiber in impotent men, prima-

Table 2-6: Causes of Veno-occlusive Dysfunction

Type	Cause
Abnormal veins	Congenital or acquired
Degeneration of tunica albuginea	Peyronie's disease, diabetes, aging, penile fracture
Alteration of erectile tissue	Smooth muscle atrophy, increased collagen deposition, alteration of endothelium or gap junction caused by aging, diabetes, or atherosclerosis
Insufficient neurotransmitter release	Psychogenic inhibition
Shunting	Congenital, traumatic, or iatrogenic shunting (eg, surgery for priapism) between corpus cavernosum and corpus spongiosum or glans

rily in patients with arteriogenic and venogenic erectile dysfunction in whom the extent of impotence corresponded with the severity of vascular disease and the failure of erectile response to papaverine injection.[28] In rabbits fed a high-cholesterol diet for 3 months, Junemann et al showed significant smooth-muscle degeneration with loss of cell-to-cell contact.[29] Cavernous nerve injury also seems to affect cavernous smooth-muscle relaxation, as demonstrated in neurotomized dogs.[30] An in vitro biochemical study showed impaired neurogenic and endothelium-related relaxation of penile smooth muscle in impotent diabetic men.[13] In vasculogenic and neurogenic erectile dysfunction, the damaged smooth muscle may be the main contributor.[31] Pickard et al also showed impairment of nerve-evoked relaxation and α-adrenergic-stimulated contraction of cavernous muscle and reduced muscle content in men with venous or mixed venous/arterial impotence.[32] In a study of cultured cavernous smooth-muscle cells, Fan et al reported an alteration of the maxi-K^+ channel in cells from impotent patients and suggested that impairment in the function or regulation of potassium channels may contribute to the decreased hyperpolarizing ability, altered calcium homeostasis, and impaired smooth-muscle relaxation in impotence.[33]

Gap junction. These intercellular communication channels can explain the synchronized and coordinated erectile response, although their pathophysiologic impact has yet to be clarified.[34] In severe arterial disease, membrane contact is lost or reduced because of the presence of large amounts of collagen fibers between cellular membranes.[35] These findings imply that a malfunction or loss of gap junctions may alter the coordinated smooth-muscle activity.

Endothelium. By releasing vasoactive agents, the endothelium of the corpora can modify the tone of adjacent smooth muscle and affect the development or inhibition of an erection. NO, prostaglandin, and the polypeptide endothelin (a strong vasoconstrictor) have been identified in the endothelial cell.[36,37] Activation of cholinergic receptors on the endothelial cell by acetylcholine and stretching of the endothelial cells as a result of increased blood flow may elicit underlying smooth-muscle relaxation through the release of NO. Diabetes and hypercholesterolemia also may alter the function of endothelium-mediated relaxation of cavernous muscle and impair erection.[38]

Most cases of veno-occlusive dysfunction represent end-organ failure and are the most difficult to treat (Table 2-6). In severe cases, the only effective treatment is penile prosthesis. Unfortunately, the pathogenesis of this end-organ failure is far from clear, and much work is required to elucidate the mechanism and pathways before effective preventive measures and restorative treatment can be designed to combat this disorder.

Drug-Induced

Various classes of therapeutic drugs can cause erectile dysfunction. For most drugs, the mechanism of action is unknown, and few well-controlled studies have examined the sexual effects of a particular drug.

Drugs that interfere with central neuroendocrine or local neurovascular control of penile smooth muscle can cause erectile dysfunction. Central neurotransmitter pathways, including 5-hydroxytryptaminergic, noradrenergic, and dopaminergic pathways involved in sexual function, may be disturbed by antipsychotics and antidepressants, as well as by some centrally acting antihypertensive drugs.

Centrally acting sympatholytics include methyldopa (Aldomet®), clonidine (Catapres®) (inhibition of the hypothalamic center via α_2-receptor stimulation), and reserpine (Serpalan®, Serpasil®) (depletion of the stores of catecholamines and serotonin). Guanethidine (Ismelin®), as a peripheral sympatholytic, has been reported to cause erectile and ejaculatory dysfunction. α-Adrenergic blocking agents such as phenoxybenzamine (Dibenzyline®) and phentolamine are also reported to cause ejaculatory inhibition. Prazosin (Minipress®), a selective α_1-adrenergic blocking agent, may cause erectile dysfunction. β-Adrenergic blockers have been reported to depress libido.[36] Thiazide diuretics have widely differing effects on potency, and spironolactone (Aldactone®) has been reported to produce erectile failure in 4% to 30% of patients and has been associated with decreased libido, gynecomastia, and mastodynia.

Major tranquilizers or antipsychotics can decrease libido, causing erectile failure and ejaculatory dysfunction. The mechanisms involved may include sedation, anticholinergic actions, a central antidopaminergic effect, α-adrenergic antagonist action, and release of prolactin. Among antidepressants, tricyclic antidepressants and monoamine oxidase (MAO) inhibitors reportedly cause erectile dysfunction through central or peripheral actions. The sexual side effects in patients taking minor tranquilizers may result from the central sedative effects of these agents.

Cigarette smoking may induce vasoconstriction and penile venous leak because of its contractile effect on cavernous smooth muscle.[24] In a study of nocturnal penile tumescence in cigarette smokers, Hirshkowitz et al reported an inverse correlation between nocturnal erection (both rigidity and duration) and the number of cigarettes smoked daily.[39] Men who smoked more than 40 cigarettes a day had the weakest and shortest nocturnal erections. Alcohol in small amounts improves erection and sex-

Psychogenic impotence: one perspective on diagnosis and treatment

Psychogenic impotence used to be a diagnosis of exclusion and assumption. Many men have experienced occasional inability to achieve or maintain erection during stress, anxiety, anger, or conflict with partner. In the 1950s and 1960s, the understanding of erectile physiology and pathophysiology was rudimentary, and no scientific test for impotence was available. When a patient complained of impotence, physicians and psychologists usually assumed that the condition was an exaggeration of a day-to-day psychological problem. This reminds me of many traditional Chinese medical books in which the terms *impotence* and *kidney failure* were interchangeable. Impotence was said to be caused by excessive masturbation, resulting in 'kidney failure.' A man was advised not to ejaculate after age 60 if he wished to live a long life. Interestingly, the Chinese blame impotence on a physical problem ('kidney failure'), while most Westerners blame it on the inner 'psyche.' To cure 'kidney failure,' traditional Chinese doctors recommended various 'tonics' made from the penises and testes of animals such as tigers, deer, and seals, as well as various herbs. In the West, several techniques (eg, sex therapy [with or without surrogate], psychoanalysis, psychotherapy) have been established to combat psychogenic impotence.

The recent success of a type V phosphodiesterase (PDE) inhibitor, sildenafil (Viagra®), in treating psychogenic impotence (sildenafil 84% vs placebo 26%) has further clouded the definition of psychogenic impotence. If, by blocking the action of PDE—an enzyme that breaks down cyclic guanine monophosphate—most psychogenically impotent patients improve their function, isn't it reasonable to assume that psychogenic impotence is just a form of neurogenic impotence at the molecular level?

ual drive because of its vasodilatory effect and the suppression of anxiety. However, large amounts can cause central sedation, decreased libido, and transient erectile dysfunction. Chronic alcoholism may also result in liver dysfunction, decreased testosterone levels, increased estrogen levels, and alcoholic polyneuropathy, which also affects penile nerves.[40] Cimetidine (Tagamet®), a histamine (H_2) receptor antagonist, has been reported to suppress libido and produce erectile failure. It is believed to act as an antiandrogen and to increase prolactin levels.[41]

Other drugs known to cause erectile dysfunction are estrogens and antiandrogens, such as ketoconazole (Nizoral®) and cyproterone acetate. Finally, many of the anticancer drugs are associated with progressive loss of libido and erectile failure. Table 2-7 lists several causes of erectile dysfunction.

Table 2-7: Diseases and Conditions Associated With Erectile Dysfunction

Disease or Condition	Cause of Erectile Dysfunction
Diabetes mellitus	Psychogenic: anxiety Neurogenic: loss of sensory and autonomic nerves Arterial: small vessel disease Venous: cavernous myopathy Endothelial dysfunction
Peyronie's disease	Loss of elasticity, penile deformity during erection Venous leak Concomitant vascular insufficiency
Aging	Decreases desire and penile sensitivity Less responsive to visual and psychological stimulation Prolongs refractory period Reduces force of emission and ejaculation
Uremia	Arterial: atherosclerosis Neurologic: peripheral neuropathy Psychological: stress and depression Medication: hypertensive medication Endocrine: hyperprolactinemia, hypogonadism, hyperparathyroidism
Smoking	Exacerbates vascular disease, resulting in arterial insufficiency and venous leak
Alcoholism	Acute: behavioral changes, CNS suppression Chronic: increases aromatization of androgens Development of peripheral neuropathy Behavioral disorder
Radiation (high dose)	Vascular insufficiency and atrophy of penile smooth muscle
AIDS	Psychogenic: depression, general weakness Neuropathy: autonomic Hormonal: defect in the hypothalamic-pituitary axis

Modified with permission from Melman A, Rehman J: Pathophysiology of erectile dysfunction. In: Vaughan ED Jr, Perlmutter AP, eds. *Atlas of Clinical Urology, Vol. 1, Impotence and Infertility.* Philadelphia, Current Medicine, 1999, pp 1.1-1.16.

Erectile Dysfunction Associated With Aging, Systemic Disease, and Other Causes

A number of studies have indicated a progressive decline in sexual function in 'healthy' aging men. Masters and Johnson noted a number of changes in older men, including greater latency to erection, less turgid erection, loss of forceful ejaculation, decreased ejaculatory volume, and a longer refractory period.[42] Decreased frequency and duration of nocturnal erection with increasing age was reported in a group of men who had regular intercourse.[43] Other research also indicates a decrease in penile tactile sensitivity with age.[16] Garban et al reported a decrease in nitric oxide synthase (NOS) activity in the penile tissue of senescent rats.[44] Christ et al suggested that a heightened cavernous muscle tone decreases erectile response in older men.[45] In one study, a decrease in testosterone in aging impotent men was associated with relatively normal gonadotropins, suggesting hypothalamic-pituitary dysfunction.[46]

Chronic renal failure has frequently been associated with diminished erectile function, impaired libido, and infertility. In one study, by the time patients with uremia began maintenance dialysis, 50% were impotent.[47] The mechanism is probably multifactorial: depressed testosterone levels, diabetes mellitus, vascular insufficiency, multiple medications, autonomic and somatic neuropathy, and psychological stress. After successful renal transplantation, 50% to 80% of patients return to their preillness potency.[48]

Patients with severe pulmonary disease often fear aggravating dyspnea during sexual intercourse. Patients with angina, heart failure, or myocardial infarction can become impotent from anxiety, depression, or arterial insufficiency. Other systemic diseases, such as liver cirrhosis, scleroderma, chronic debilitation, and cachexia, can also cause erectile dysfunction.

The penis is a specialized blood vessel under the control of its master's mind, nerves, and hormone level. Any condition that affects the master's mind, hormonal balance, nervous system, or circulatory system can adversely affect the penile erection. The physician should not just brush aside a patient's complaint of erectile dysfunction as a psychological problem or an old man's dream of regaining youth. Instead, clinicians should be aware that most of these complaints are linked to physical causes, and a positive attitude should be taken toward detecting the causes and treating the patient's 'mind and body' accordingly.

References

1. NIH Consensus Conference: Impotence. NIH Consensus Development Panel on Impotence. *JAMA* 1993; 270:83-90.

2. Kinsey AC, Pomeroy WB, Martin CE: *Sexual Behavior in the Human Male.* Philadelphia, WB Saunders, 1948, p 236.

3. Diokno AC, Brown MB, Herzog AR: Sexual function in the elderly. *Arch Intern Med* 1990;150:197-200.

4. Feldman HA, Goldstein I, Hatzichristou DG, et al: Impotence and its medical and psychosocial correlates: results of the Massachusetts Male Aging Study. *J Urol* 1994;151:54-61.

5. Masters WH, Johnson V: *Human Sexual Response.* Boston, Little Brown & Co, 1970.

6. Eardley I, Kirby RS: Neurogenic impotence. In: Kirby RS, Carson CC,

Webster GD, eds. *Impotence: Diagnosis and Management of Male Erectile Dysfunction*. Boston, Butterworth-Heinemann, 1991, pp 227-231.

7. Courtois FJ, Macdougall JC, Sachs BD: Erectile mechanism in paraplegia. *Physiol Behav* 1993;53:721-726.

8. Finkle AL, Taylor SP: Sexual potency after radical prostatectomy. *J Urol* 1981;125:350-352.

9. Veenema RJ, Gursel EO, Lattimer JK: Radical retropubic prostatectomy for cancer: a 20-year experience. *J Urol* 1977; 117:330-331.

10. Weinstein M, Roberts M: Sexual potency following surgery for rectal carcinoma. A followup of 44 patients. *Ann Surg* 1977;185:295-300.

11. Walsh PC, Donker PJ: Impotence following radical prostatectomy: insight into etiology and prevention. *J Urol* 1982; 128:492-497.

12. Catalona WJ, Bigg SW: Nerve-sparing radical prostatectomy: evaluation of results after 250 patients. *J Urol* 1990; 143:538-544.

13. Saenz de Tejada I, Goldstein I, Azadzoi K, et al: Impaired neurogenic and endothelium-mediated relaxation of penile smooth muscle from diabetic men with impotence. *N Engl J Med* 1989;320:1025-1030.

14. Brock G, Nunes L, Padma-Nathan H, et al: Nitric oxide synthase: a new diagnostic tool for neurogenic impotence. *Urology* 1993;42:412-417.

15. Bemelmans BL, Meuleman EJ, Anten BW, et al: Penile sensory disorders in erectile dysfunction: results of comprehensive neuro-urophysiological diagnostic evaluation in 123 patients. *J Urol* 1991;146:777-782.

16. Rowland DL, Greenleaf W, Mas M, et al: Penile and finger sensory thresholds in young, aging, and diabetic males. *Arch Sex Behav* 1989;18:1-12.

17. Cunningham GR, Hirshkowitz M, Korenman SG, et al: Testosterone replacement therapy and sleep-related erections in hypogonadal men. *J Clin Endocrinol Metab* 1990;70:792-797.

18. Bancroft J, Wu FC: Changes in erectile responsiveness during androgen replacement therapy. *Arch Sex Behav* 1983; 12:59-66.

19. Graham CW, Regan JB: Blinded clinical trial of testosterone enanthate in impotent men with low or low-normal serum testosterone levels. *Int J Impot Res* 1992;4:P144.

20. Leonard MP, Nickel CJ, Morales A: Hyperprolactinemia and impotence: why, when and how to investigate. *J Urol* 1989; 142:992-994.

21. Michal V, Ruzbarsky V: Histological changes in the penile arterial bed with aging and diabetes. In: Zorgniotti AW, Rossi G, eds. *Vasculogenic Impotence: Proceedings of the First International Conference on Corpus Cavernosum Revascularization*. Springfield, IL, Charles C. Thomas, 1980, pp 113-119.

22. Goldstein I, Feldman MI, Deckers PJ, et al: Radiation-associated impotence. A clinical study of its mechanism. *JAMA* 1984;251:903-910.

23. Levine FJ, Greenfield AJ, Goldstein I: Arteriographically determined occlusive disease within the hypogastric-cavernous bed in impotent patients following blunt perineal and pelvic trauma. *J Urol* 1990; 144:1147-1153.

24. Junemann KP, Lue TF, Luo JA, et al: The effect of cigarette smoking on penile erection. *J Urol* 1987;138:438-441.

25. Rosen MP, Greenfield AJ, Walker TG, et al: Arteriogenic impotence: findings in 195 impotent men examined with selective internal pudendal angiography. Young Investigator's Award. *Radiology* 1990;174:1043-1048.

26. Hsieh JT, Muller SC, Lue TF: The influence of blood flow and blood pressure on penile erection. *Int J Impot Res* 1989;1:35-42.

27. Cerami A, Vlassara H, Brownlee M: Glucose and aging. *Sci Am* 1987;256: 90-96.

28. Wespes E, Goes PM, Schiffmann S, et al: Computerized analysis of smooth muscle fibers in potent and impotent patients. *J Urol* 1991;146:1015-1017.

29. Junemann KP, Aufenanger J, Konrad T, et al: The effect of impaired lipid metabolism on the smooth muscle cells of rabbits. *Urol Res* 1991;19:271-275.

30. Paick JS, Goldsmith PC, Batra AK, et al: Relationship between venous incompetence and cavernous nerve injury: ultrastructural alteration of cavernous smooth muscle in the neurotomized dog. *Int J Impot Res* 1991;3:185-195.

31. Mersdorf A, Goldsmith PC, Diederichs W, et al: Ultrastructural changes in impotent penile tissue: a comparison of 65 patients. *J Urol* 1991; 145:749-758.

32. Pickard RS, Powell PH, Zar MA: The effect of inhibitors of nitric oxide biosynthesis and cyclic GMP formation on nerve-evoked relaxation of human cavernosal smooth muscle. *Br J Pharmacol* 1991;104:755-759.

33. Fan SF, Brink PR, Melman A, et al: An analysis of the Maxi-K+ (KCa) channel in cultured human corporal smooth muscle cells. *J Urol* 1995; 153:818-825.

34. Christ GJ, Moreno AP, Parker ME, et al: Intercellular communication through gap junctions: a potential role in pharmacomechanical coupling and syncytial tissue contraction in vascular smooth muscle isolated from the human corpus cavernosum. *Life Sci* 1991;49:PL195-PL200.

35. Persson C, Diederichs W, Lue TF, et al: Correlation of altered penile ultrastructure with clinical arterial evaluation. *J Urol* 1989;142:1462-1468.

36. Ignarro LJ, Bush PA, Buga GM, et al: Neurotransmitter identity doubt. *Nature* 1990;347:131-132.

37. Saenz de Tejada I, Carson MP, de las Morenas A, et al: Endothelin: localization, synthesis, activity, and receptor types in human penile corpus cavernosum. *Am J Physiol* 1991;261:H1078-H1085.

38. Wein AJ, Van Arsdalen KN: Drug-induced male sexual dysfunction. *Urol Clin North Am* 1988;15:23-31.

39. Hirshkowitz M, Karacan I, Howell JW, et al: Nocturnal penile tumescence in cigarette smokers with erectile dysfunction. *Urology* 1992;39:101-107.

40. Miller NS, Gold MS: The human sexual response and alcohol and drugs. *J Subst Abuse Treat* 1988;5:171-177.

41. Wolfe MM: Impotence of cimetidine treatment. *N Engl J Med* 1979;300:94.

42. Masters WH, Johnson VE: Sex after sixty-five. *Reflections* 1977;12:31-43.

43. Schiavi RC, Schreiner-Engel P: Nocturnal penile tumescence in healthy aging men. *J Gerontol* 1988;43:M146-M150.

44. Garban H, Vernet D, Freedman A, et al: Effect of aging on nitric oxide-mediated penile erection in rats. *Am J Physiol* 1995;268:H467-H475.

45. Christ GJ, Maayani S, Valcic M, et al: Pharmacological studies of human erectile tissue: characteristics of spontaneous contractions and alterations in alpha-adrenoceptor responsiveness with age and disease in isolated tissues. *Br J Pharmacol* 1990;101:375-381.

46. Kaiser FE, Viosca SP, Morley JE, et al: Impotence and aging: clinical and hormonal factors. *J Am Geriatr Soc* 1988;36:511-519.

47. David KR, Koyle M: Impotence in chronic renal failure. In: Rajfer Y, ed. *Common Problems in Infertility and Impotence*. Chicago, Year Book Medical Publishers, 1990, pp 368-375.

48. Salvatierra O Jr, Fortmann JL, Belzer FO: Sexual function of males before and after renal transplantation. *Urology* 1975; 5:64-66.

Chapter 3

History, Physical Examination, and Laboratory Tests

The therapeutic strategy of treating male impotence is to correct the cause of impotence or to bypass the cause and offer a nonspecific treatment. The ultimate goal is to convert the sexually and mentally crippled patient and his frustrated partner to a satisfied, sexually practicing couple. Since the introduction of sildenafil (Viagra®) in 1998, many men have obtained the drug without seeing a physician (such as through Internet pharmacies). We believe it is in the patient's best interest that a detailed work-up is performed to find the underlying cause.

According to the American Heritage Dictionary, *diagnosis* is defined as "(a) the act or process of identifying or determining the nature and cause of a disease or injury through evaluation of patient history, examination, and review of laboratory data; (b) the opinion derived from such an evaluation." The physician must identify the cause of disease and treat accordingly. Some of the most effective treatments for erectile dysfunction are nonspecific and are useful for all types of impotence. Clinicians may attempt to treat without an appropriate work-up. On the other hand, sophisticated tests are now available, especially for neuro-

genic and vasculogenic impotence, and the added cost can be substantial if every patient is offered these tests.

We have used the patient's goal-directed approach[1] (Figure 3-1) for the past 10 years. We recommend that every patient undergo a thorough medical and psychosexual history, a detailed physical examination, and appropriate laboratory tests so that potentially life-threatening causes can be detected. Further diagnostic testing is tailored to the treatment chosen by the patient. The physician also should consider the patient's profile: age, general health, concomitant medical disease, the goals and expectations of the patient and his partner, etc. Then the physician and patient together can decide the next diagnostic or therapeutic step. A variety of treatment options is available. Our diagnostic approach for each treatment option is listed in Table 3-1.

Medical and Psychosexual History

Despite the explosion of new diagnostic tests, a detailed psychosexual and medical history remains the key to diagnosis of erectile dysfunction. A detailed history also helps differentiate erectile failure from changes in li-

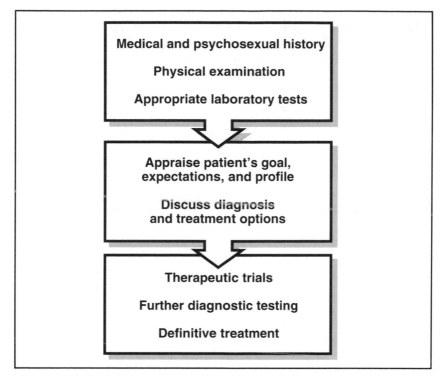

Figure 3-1: Patient's goal-directed approach to diagnosis and treatment of erectile dysfunction.

bido, orgasm, and ejaculation. Because of the sensitive nature of this discussion, the physician must establish early on a relationship of trust with the patient.

A careful medical history should include concurrent illnesses and medications. Because erectile dysfunction may have multiple causes, a detailed history and physical examination may help determine whether the dysfunction results from anatomic, endocrinologic, neurologic, vascular, or psychogenic abnormalities.

The psychosexual history should include quality of erection, duration of impotence, level of libido, and a complete inventory of sexual partners. An assessment of the onset of dysfunction, the presence of morning erection, and any psychological conflict may help determine whether the dysfunction is primarily psychogenic or organic (Table 3-2). The sexual history often provides the most helpful information in directing further evaluation and treatment. For example, a patient who reports a recent history of impotence associated with low libido may suffer from an endocrinopathy that can be easily treated with hormone replacement.

A psychogenic disorder occasionally is the primary cause of erectile dysfunction. Early recognition avoids unnecessary and often costly diagnostic tests. Because erectile dysfunction

Table 3-1: Diagnostic Tests for Chosen Treatment Options*

Treatment Options	Diagnostic Tests
Oral, topical, or intraurethral medication; vacuum constriction device	None (CIS or duplex ultrasound [optional])
Intracavernous injection	CIS (duplex ultrasound optional)
Penile prosthesis	NPT (RigiScan®) or CIS or duplex ultrasound
Venous surgery	CIS + duplex ultrasound + cavernosography (or DICC) + NPT
Arterial surgery	CIS + duplex ultrasound (or DICC) + arteriography (NPT optional)

* Additional testing to be undertaken after complete history, physical examination, and laboratory testing

CIS = combined intracavernous injection and stimulation test, DICC = dynamic infusion cavernosometry and cavernosography, NPT = nocturnal penile tumescence

Used with permission from Walsh PC, Retik AB, Vaughan ED Jr, et al, eds: *Campbell's Urology*, 7th ed. Philadelphia, WB Saunders, 1997, chapter 39.

Table 3-2: Differentiation Between Psychogenic and Organic Impotence

Characteristic	Organic	Psychogenic
Onset	Gradual	Acute
Circumstances	Global	Situational
Course	Constant	Varying
Noncoital erection	Poor	Rigid
Psychosexual problem	Secondary	Long history
Partner problem	Secondary	At onset
Anxiety and fear	Secondary	Primary

Modified from Hengeveld MW: Erectile disorder: a psychosexological review. In: Jonas U, Thon WF, Stief CG, eds. *Erectile Dysfunction*. Berlin, Springer-Verlag, 1991. Used with permission.

Table 3-3: Common Physical Signs in Various Types of Impotence

Types of Impotence	Common Physical Signs
Psychogenic	Anxiety, unease, restlessness, denial
Hormonal	
• thyroid	Enlarged thyroid, exophthalmos
• testes	Gynecomastia, loss of body hair, atrophic or absent testes
• pituitary	Impaired visual field
Neurogenic	Decreased genital and perineal sensation, absent bulbocavernosus reflex, weakness of extremities
Arterial	Decreased femoral or pedal pulses
Cavernosal	Peyronie's plaque, micropenis

is associated with many common medical conditions and medications, careful questioning may yield clues. A history of peripheral vascular or coronary arterial disease, diabetes, renal failure, tobacco and alcohol use, or neurologic or chronic debilitating disease can direct further evaluation. Older patients with a long history of diabetes and vascular disease are likely to have impotence secondary to vascular and neuropathic disease. On the other hand, young patients with psychiatric illness are more likely to have psychogenic impotence or impotence secondary to psychotropic medications. Neuroleptic treatment can restore desire but may cause erectile, orgasmic, and sexual satisfaction problems. Surgical history may yield similar insights. Radical pelvic surgery (eg, prostatectomy, abdominoperineal resection), radiation, and pel-

vic trauma are well known to be associated with impotence.[2,3]

Physical Examination

A thorough physical examination with particular attention to sexual and genital development may occasionally reveal an obvious cause (eg, micropenis, chordee, Peyronie's disease) (Table 3-3). The finding of small, soft, atrophic testes or gynecomastia should prompt an endocrine evaluation for hypogonadism or hyperprolactinemia. Patients with certain genetic syndromes, such as Kallmann's syndrome or Klinefelter's syndrome, may present with obvious physical signs of hypogonadism or a distinctive body habitus. A careful neurologic examination should also be performed. Testing for genital and perineal sensation and the bulbocavernosus reflex also is useful in assessing possible neurogenic impotence. Signs of thy-

Table 3-4: Treatment Options for Erectile Dysfunction: Costs, Advantages, and Disadvantages

Treatment	Cost ($)	Advantages	Disadvantages/ Side Effects
Psychosexual therapy	75-200/session	Noninvasive; moderately successful therapy resolves conflict	High recurrence rate
Oral drugs*	1-3/day	Noninvasive	Poor efficacy; frequent systemic side effects
Sildenafil (Viagra®)	9-10 per 100 mg dose	Noninvasive	Systemic side effects
Tadalafil (Cialis®)	9-10 per 20 mg dose	Noninvasive	Systemic side effects
Vardenafil (Levitra®)	9-10 per 20 mg dose	Noninvasive	Systemic side effects
Vacuum constriction device	150-550/device	Low cost, noninvasive	Unnatural erection; petechiae, pain
Transurethral therapy	25/dose	Minimally invasive	Lower success rate than injection; penile pain
Intracavernous injection	5-25/dose	Natural erection, highly successful	More invasive; priapism, fibrosis, pain
Prosthesis	6,000-15,000	Highly successful	Requires surgery, anesthesia; infection, fibrosis
Vascular surgery	8,000-15,000	Restores natural erection	Moderate success rate; requires surgery, anesthesia

* Drugs other than sildenafil, tadalafil, and vardenafil.
Used with permission from Walsh PC, Retik AB, Vaughan ED Jr, et al, eds: *Campbell's Urology*, 7th ed. Philadelphia, WB Saunders, 1997, chapter 39.

roid underactivity or overactivity should be explored, as well as stigmata of liver failure, renal failure, or anemia. Hypertension and cardiac arrhythmia should also be assessed (Table 3-3).

Davis-Joseph et al reported that history and physical examination had a 95% sensitivity but only a 50% specificity in diagnosing organic erectile dysfunction, and they concluded that a multifaceted comprehensive approach is required for a definitive diagnosis of erectile dysfunction.[4] In many cases, a careful medical and psychosexual history and physical examination directs the physician to the most expedient and cost-effective approach and eliminates the need for unnecessary diagnostic tests.

Laboratory Investigation

The laboratory investigation is directed at identifying treatable conditions or previously undetected medical illnesses that may contribute to erectile dysfunction, such as metabolic disturbances or endocrine abnormalities. A basic laboratory evaluation includes complete blood count, urinalysis, renal and liver function, lipid profile, and morning testosterone.

Discussion of the Available Options

Informing the patient and partner of the available diagnostic and therapeutic options is an important aspect of the office consultation. Treatment options and their costs, advantages, and disadvantages are listed in Table 3-4.

In the late 1970s and early 1980s, the penile prosthesis and psychosexual therapy were the only two effective treatments for erectile dysfunction. The introductions of the less invasive but highly effective intracavernous injection and vacuum constriction device and, more recently, transurethral therapy and new oral medication have dramatically changed management. The success of these nonspecific treatments has led many physicians to question the wisdom of the traditional medical approach of making an accurate diagnosis and following up with specific treatment. Although finding and correcting the exact cause seems to be the most logical approach, the current socioeconomic climate argues strongly against it. Therefore, we propose the patient's goal-directed approach, which determines the extent of further work-up according to the patient's age, general health, and treatment goal.

References

1.   Lue TF: Impotence: a patient's goal-directed approach to treatment. *World J Urol* 1990;8:67.

2.   Armenakas NA, McAninch JW, Lue TF, et al: Posttraumatic impotence: magnetic resonance imaging and duplex ultrasound in diagnosis and management. *J Urol* 1993;149:1272-1275.

3.   Walsh PC, Partin AW, Epstein JI: Cancer control and quality of life following anatomical radical retropubic prostatectomy: results at 10 years. *J Urol* 1994; 152:1831-1836.

4.   Davis-Joseph B, Tiefer L, Melman A: Accuracy of the initial history and physical examination to establish the etiology of erectile dysfunction. *Urology* 1995;45:498-502.

Chapter 4

Additional Investigations

*In France in the 16th and 17th centuries, up to 2,000 legal judge-
ments were made in cases of impotence as the basis for annulment
of marriage. The lengthy procedure was divided into five stages.
The first was the husband's confession. The second was a neighbor-
hood inquiry. The third was a 3-year trial period. The fourth was
cross-examination by judges, and genital examination of husband
and wife by surgeons and matrons. The final stage was the Test of
Congress: a public display of the consummation of the sexual act in
the presence of doctors, surgeons, matrons, and judges.—Brenot[1]*

In addition to a history, physical examination, and laboratory tests, some patients may choose to try medications or devices, while others may desire a more detailed investigation to identify the cause of erectile dysfunction. This chapter reviews the more sophisticated tests for various causes of erectile dysfunction.

Nocturnal Penile Tumescence Testing

Nocturnal penile tumescence (NPT), or sleep-related erection, is a recurring cycle of penile erections associated with REM sleep in almost all potent men. In 1970, Karacan suggested that NPT could be used to evaluate erectile dysfunction because its mechanism presumably relies on neurovascular responses similar to those of erotically induced erections.[2] The primary goal of NPT testing is to distinguish between psychogenic and organic causes of impotence.

Although NPT testing is noninvasive, its clinical usefulness has been questioned. Anxiety and depression can sometimes influence the content of the dream state, negatively affecting spontaneous nocturnal erections. Additionally, sleep disturbances such as apnea and motor agitation can induce erroneous recordings. Dysfunction at the level of the cortex and spine may still permit nocturnal tumescence while causing an erectile deficit when awake. Moreover, normal NPT may occur in patients with mild vascular problems (such as 'pelvic steal syndrome') who often lose erection during pelvic thrusts. All these factors question the clinical effectiveness of the NPT test in the study of the cause of impotence. Moreover, NPT evaluation is expensive ($1,500 to $3,500) because it often is done in a specially equipped sleep center.

The RigiScan® was introduced in 1985. This combines the sophisticated monitoring of rigidity, tumescence, and number and duration of events with the convenience and economic advantage of an ambulatory monitoring system.[3] Normative data supplied by Timm Medical describe three to six

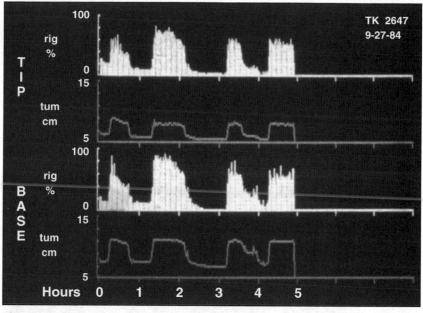

Figure 4-1: RigiScan® result of a 35-year-old with four episodes of good erections during a 5-hour sleep. (Courtesy of Timm Medical.)

erection episodes, each lasting 10 to 15 minutes per 8-hour sleep, with at least one erection with a circumference increase of >3 cm at the base and >2 cm at the tip, sustained for at least 10 minutes at a rigidity >70% (Figures 4-1 and 4-2). A new software program that summarizes an entire night of tumescence and rigidity data into a single value is available, giving the rigidity activity unit (RAU) and tumescence activity unit (TAU) on a nomogram.[4]

Many investigators have advocated the use of NPT studies, particularly in patients with psychogenic impotence.[5] A normal finding in a patient in whom a psychologic cause is suspected may help reduce the cost of evaluation by avoiding unnecessary endocrine and vascular evaluation. However, because of the problems associated with

---

Table 4-1: Indications for Nocturnal Penile Tumescence Testing

Medical	To confirm psychogenic impotence before psychosexual therapy
	To rule out psychogenic impotence before surgical intervention
	As a research tool for clinical studies
Medicolegal	To help differentiate psychogenic from organic impotence

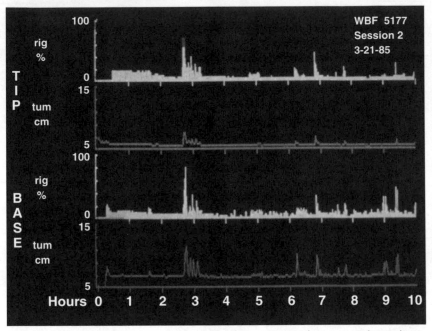

Figure 4-2: A man with several poor-rigidity erections during an 8-hour sleep. (Courtesy of Timm Medical.)

various NPT tests, findings often need to be independently confirmed by other studies. For these reasons, we have abandoned NPT testing as a routine part of the impotence evaluation. However, in some selected cases (eg, patients with complex and confusing histories, those involved in litigation in which compensation or guilt hinges on erectile status[6]), we agree that NPT is useful in confirming clinical diagnosis (Table 4-1). In these cases, for financial reasons, we begin with a RigiScan® test because a normal result rules out significant vascular insufficiency. When abnormal NPT is noted on Rigi-Scan® and the clinical diagnosis is uncertain, a formal sleep laboratory study with polysomnography (Table 4-2) may be indicated to rule out sleep apnea and nocturnal myoclonus as the cause of impaired erection. Table 4-3 lists conditions that adversely affect the accuracy of NPT results.

Psychometry and Psychological Interview

For most patients, a detailed psychosexual history is the only requirement before proceeding to treatment. However, in some men, deep-seated psychological or psychiatric problems seem to be the primary cause of sexual difficulty. In these cases, a psychological or psychiatric consultation is advised. Several psychometric instruments are available for the evaluation of erectile dysfunction: (1) standardized personality questionnaires, (2) the depression inventory, and (3) questionnaires for sexual dysfunction and relationship factors. A skillful diagnostic interview

Table 4-2: Contemporary Polysomnographic Recording Montage[6]

Central Electroencephalography (EEG)

Electro-oculography (EOG)

Submental Electromyography (EMG)

Sleep-Related Cardiopulmonary Function
- Nasal/oral airflow thermography
- Abdominal movement
- Pulse oximetry recorded from ear
- Heart rate and rhythm

Limb Movement
- Left and right anterior tibialis EMG

Sleep-Related Erections
- Circumference change at penile base and tip (coronal sulcus)
- Segmental pulsatile blood flow (optional)
- Bulbocavernous/ischiocavernous muscle activity (optional)

Used with permission from Walsh PC, Retik AB, Vaughan ED Jr, et al, eds: *Campbell's Urology*, 7th ed. Philadelphia, WB Saunders, 1997, chapter 39.

remains the mainstay of psychological evaluation. Traditional psychoanalytic theory has been replaced by a newer concept popularized by Kaplan, who theorizes that the determinants of psychogenic impotence operate on different levels of causation, ranging from superficial and mild problems to those deeply rooted in early life.[7] Hartmann suggests that the interview should be focused on the following: (1) the current sexual problem and its history, (2) deeper causes of sexual dysfunction, (3) the relationship (dyadic causes), and (4) psychiatric symptoms.[8]

In obtaining the sexual history, the interviewer should strive to determine whether the dysfunction is primary or secondary; constant, phasic, or situational; and partner-specific. The interviewer should also determine the degree of noncoital erections (masturbatory, nocturnal, or morning) and the patient's history of trauma, cultural or educational indoctrination, and neurotic processes in which sexual symptoms may defend against unconscious fear. In assessing a partner-related problem, the couple should be interviewed together and apart, if possible.

Although psychological consultation is not indicated for most patients with nonpsychogenic causes of erectile dysfunction, it is useful in directing treatment in patients with deep-

Table 4-3: Conditions That May Contribute to False-Negative or False-Positive NPT (10%-20%)

False-Positive NPT

- Neurogenic impotence, especially sensory or incomplete lesions
- Pelvic steal syndrome
- Mild vascular or neurologic insufficiency

False-Negative NPT

- Sleep disorders (eg, sleep apnea, nocturnal myoclonus)
- Significant anxiety and depression
- Hypogonadism
- Febrile disease
- Healthy elderly patient (less duration, frequency, and rigidity)
- Drugs (eg, alcohol, tobacco, antiandrogens, antidepressants, marijuana, narcotics)

NPT = nocturnal penile tumescence

Modified with permission from Melman A, Rehman J: Pathophysiology of erectile dysfunction. In: Vaughan ED Jr, Perlmutter AP, eds. *Atlas of Clinical Urology, Vol. 1, Impotence and Infertility.* Philadelphia, Current Medicine, 1999, pp 1.1-1.16.

seated psychological problems. For example, a patient with severe depression, a strained relationship, or unrealistic expectations will likely not enjoy a satisfactory outcome, even with a perfectly functioning penile prosthesis.

Neurologic Testing

In a broader sense, neurologic testing should assess peripheral, spinal, and supraspinal centers and both somatic and autonomic pathways. However, the effect of neurologic deficit on penile erection is complicated, and, with few exceptions, neurologic testing rarely changes management. Moreover, no reliable test exists to assess neurotransmitter release, which leaves a significant

gap in the overall assessment of neurologic function associated with penile erection. Neurologic testing aims to (1) uncover reversible neurologic disease such as dorsal nerve neuropathy secondary to long-distance bicycling; (2) assess the extent of neurologic deficit from a known neurologic disease, such as diabetes mellitus or pelvic injury; and (3) determine whether referral to a neurologist is necessary (eg, work-up for possible spinal cord tumor).

Somatic Nervous System

Biothesiometry. This test measures the sensory perception threshold to various amplitudes of vibratory stimulation produced by a handheld electromagnetic device (biothesiometer) placed on the

Table 4-4: Penile Biothesiometry[9]

Age Range (years)	Right Finger	Left Finger	Right Shaft	Left Shaft	Glans
17-29	5	5	5	5	6
30-39	5	5	6	6	7
40-49	5	5	6	6	7
50-59	6	6	8	8	9
60-69	6	6	9	9	10
Older than 70	7	7	14	14	16

* Numbers represent average vibration threshold to nearest whole number in potent control subjects with no neuropathology.

Used with permission from Walsh PC, Retik AB, Vaughan ED Jr, et al, eds: *Campbell's Urology*, 7th ed. Philadelphia, WB Saunders, 1997, chapter 39.

pulp of the index fingers, both sides of the penile shaft, and the glans penis.[9] Although some argue that it cannot replace neurophysiologic tests, many urologists use this test as an office screening (Table 4-4) to select patients for neurologic consultation.

Sacral evoked response—bulbocavernosus reflex latency. This test is performed by placing two stimulating ring electrodes around the penis, one near the corona and the other 3 cm proximal. Concentric needle electrodes are placed in the right and left bulbocavernous muscles to record the response. Square-wave impulses are delivered by a direct current stimulator. The latency period for each stimulus response is measured from the beginning of the stimulus to the beginning of the response. An abnormal bulbocavernosus reflex (BCR) latency time, defined as more than three standard deviations above the mean (30 to 40 msec), indicates a high probability of neuropathology.[10]

Dorsal nerve conduction velocity. In patients with adequate penile length, two BCR latency measurements can be made, one from the glans and one from the base of the penis, to determine the conduction velocity of the dorsal nerve. Gerstenberg and Bradley determined an average conduction velocity of 23.5 m/sec with a range of 21.4 to 29.1 m/sec in normal subjects.[11]

Genitocerebral evoked-potential studies. This test involves electric stimulation of the dorsal nerve of the penis as described for the BCR latency test. Instead of recording electromyographic (EMG) responses, this study records the evoked-potential waveforms overlying the sacral spinal cord and cerebral cortex.[9] This study objectively assesses the presence, location, and nature of afferent penile sensory dysfunction.

Autonomic Nervous System

Heart rate variability and sympathetic skin response. Although autonomic neuropathy is an important cause of erectile dysfunction, direct testing is not available. Tests of heart rate control and blood pressure control are indirect methods of assessment. Because heart rate and blood pressure responses can be affected by many external factors, these tests must be done under standardized conditions.[12]

Smooth-muscle EMG and single-potential analysis of cavernous electric activity. Direct recording of cavernous electric activity with a needle electrode during flaccidity and with visual sexual stimulation was first reported by Wagner et al.[13] Stief et al reported that, in normal subjects, single-potential analysis of cavernous electric activity (SPACE) shows a regular pattern of activity with long phases of electric silence at the usual amplification interrupted by synchronous, low-frequency, high-amplitude potentials.[14] In patients with disruption of the peripheral autonomic supply, asynchronous potentials with higher frequencies and an irregular shape are typical. In those with complete spinal cord lesions, abnormal and normal electric activity are found. More studies are needed to define the clinical utility of SPACE.

Hormonal Assessment

Endocrinopathy leading to impotence may be a manifestation of a more serious, possibly life-threatening disease, such as a prolactin-secreting tumor.[15] For these reasons, some urologists routinely measure testosterone and prolactin levels in initial evaluation. Because testosterone-binding globulin (TeBG) is decreased in hypothyroidism, obesity, and acromegaly and increased in hyperthyroidism and estrogen therapy, the free biologically active hormone must be measured in these conditions when total testosterone can be misleading. In men, testosterone secretion occurs episodically with a diurnal rhythm. The highest level occurs in the early morning, followed by a progressive decrease to the lowest level in the evening. The high and low levels may differ by 30%. For practical reasons, we usually obtain a single measurement of morning testosterone (normal, 300 to 1,000 ng/dL). If the result is abnormal, we repeat the test and obtain levels of prolactin, luteinizing hormone (LH) (normal, 1 to 15 mIU/mL) and follicle-stimulating hormone (FSH) (normal, 1 to 15 mIU/mL) to differentiate primary from secondary hypogonadism. Only men with clearly documented hypogonadism are candidates for testosterone replacement therapy. We refer patients with secondary hypogonadism to an endocrinologist for further work-up of possible pituitary or hypothalamic dysfunction.

Abnormally elevated prolactin levels (>22 ng/mL) can lower testosterone secretion through inhibition of LH-releasing hormone (LHRH) secretion by the hypothalamus, resulting in impotence. Although the incidence of prolactin-secreting tumor is extremely low, a high percentage of these patients (>90%) will have impotence and decreased libido as the presenting complaint.[15] Hyperprolactinemia may also be caused by certain drugs or medical conditions such as renal insufficiency and hypothyroidism or may be idiopathic.

Some men with gynecomastia or suspected androgen resistance (high serum testosterone and LH with undermasculinization) should undergo determination of serum estradiol and androgen receptors on the genital skin. Patients with a rapid loss of secondary sex characteristics may have testicular and adrenal failure and should also be tested for adrenal function.[16] Other endocrine disorders, such as hyperthyroidism and hypothyroidism and adrenocortical dysfunction or tumor, may affect sexual function and should be investigated if suspected.

Vascular Evaluation
Penile Brachial Pressure Index

The penile brachial index (PBI) represents the penile systolic blood pressure divided by the brachial systolic blood pressure. A penile brachial index of 0.7 or less indicates arteriogenic impotence.[17] However, this test has many limitations: (1) measurement in the flaccid state does not reveal the full functional capacity of the cavernous arteries in the erect state; and (2) the continuous-wave Doppler probe does not discriminately select the arterial flow of the paired cavernous arteries, because the probe detects all pulsatile flow within its path and usually detects the higher blood flow of the dorsal penile artery, which is located superficially. Therefore, a normal PBI cannot be relied on to exclude arteriogenic impotence.

Combined Intracavernous Injection and Stimulation Test

Differentiation among psychogenic, neurogenic, and vascular causes is often difficult, even after obtaining a detailed history, physical examination, and endocrine evaluation. Additional information about the vascular status of the penis often helps. Intracorporeal injection of papaverine, first introduced by Virag et al,[18] was found to be a useful, inexpensive, and minimally invasive diagnostic tool in patients with suspected vasculogenic impotence.[18,19] The pharmacologic screening test allows the clinician to bypass neurogenic and hormonal influences and to directly and objectively evaluate the vascular status of the penis.

We currently use papaverine (30 mg), papaverine + phentolamine (0.3 mL), or alprostadil (10 µg) for the test. The medication is injected into the corpus cavernosum through an insulin or tuberculin syringe with a 28-gauge, 5/8-inch needle. The erectile response is periodically evaluated for rigidity and duration. Full erection (ie, an erection >90° and firm to palpation) normally is achieved within 15 minutes and lasts longer than 15 minutes.[20]

A normal finding rules out the possibility of venous leak, although about 20% of patients with arterial insufficiency may achieve a rigid erection because of an intact veno-occlusive mechanism.[21] An abnormal pharmacologic test result suggests penile vascular disease (eg, arterial, venous, cavernous) and warrants further evaluation, although it may not always be indicative.[20] Patients' fear of injection often produces a heightened sympathetic response, which may produce a false-positive result. To obtain better results, patients also are instructed to perform self-stimulation if a rigid erection does not occur within 15 minutes. This technique

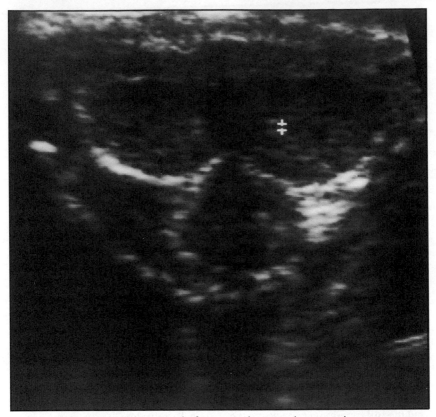

Figure 4-3: Duplex ultrasound of a penis showing the paired corpora cavernosa, the corpus spongiosum, and the two cavernous arteries. The diameters of the arteries can be measured as indicated.

is the combined injection and stimulation (CIS) test. In our experience, many patients (about 75%) who initially have a subnormal response to intracavernous injection will have significant improvement in their erections after self-stimulation.[22]

Duplex Ultrasonography (Gray-Scale and Color-Coded)

Duplex sonography provides clear advantages over previous techniques. First, in contrast to pudendal arteriography, duplex sonography is noninvasive and can be performed in the office setting. Second, the high-resolution duplex ultrasound probe allows the ultrasonographer to selectively image the individual cavernous arteries and perform Doppler blood flow analysis simultaneously within these vessels.[23] The color-coded Doppler device provides an additional advantage of easier assessment of direction of blood flow and communication among the cavernous, dorsal, and spongiosal arteries, which are crucial in penile vascular and reconstructive surgery.

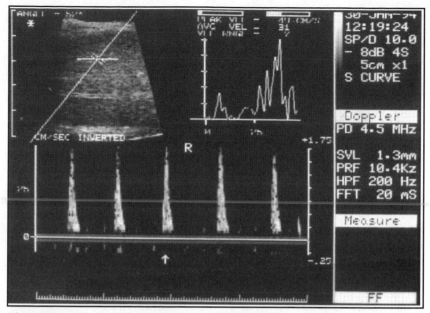

Figure 4-4: Duplex ultrasound shows the cursor was placed on the right cavernous artery. Peak flow velocity was 49 cm/sec, indicating a good arterial flow.

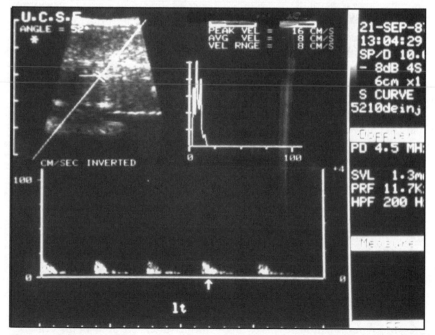

Figure 4-5: A peak flow velocity of 16 cm/sec, indicating a poor arterial flow.

The study is performed by first obtaining a baseline anatomic study of the flaccid penis. The arterial diameter of the flaccid penis and the presence of any calcification within the vessel wall are noted.

A pharmacologic erection is then induced by intracavernous injection of one of the following: papaverine (30 mg), papaverine + phentolamine (0.3 mL), or alprostadil (10 µg). Sonographic assessment of the penis is then repeated 3 to 5 minutes after the injection. Each main cavernous and dorsal artery is individually assessed. Cavernous arterial diameter and pulsation are recorded. The presence of communication between the paired cavernous arteries or among the dorsal, spongiosal, and cavernous arteries also should be noted. An asymmetric response of the cavernous arteries, a thickened arterial wall, or the lack of arterial pulsation may indicate a significant lesion.[24] We encourage all patients to perform manual self-stimulation in a private setting. Scanning is then repeated and, if necessary, repeated again after a second injection and self-stimulation.

The normal Doppler response is a peak systolic flow velocity of more than 30 cm/sec in both cavernous arteries and a strong phasic pulsation with diameter change between systolic and diastolic phases (Figures 4-3, 4-4, and 4-5). Adequate veno-occlusive mechanism is characterized by a sustained rigid erection and an absence of end-diastolic flow 20 minutes after injection.

Cavernous Arterial Occlusion Pressure

This variation of penile blood pressure determination involves injection of vasodilators (usually 30 mg papaverine + 2 mg phentolamine) followed by infusion of saline solution into the corpora cavernosa at a rate sufficient to raise the intracavernous pressure above the systolic blood pressure. A Doppler transducer is then applied to the side of the penile base. The saline infusion is stopped, and the intracavernous pressure is allowed to fall. The pressure at which the cavernous arterial flow becomes detectable is the cavernous artery systolic occlusion pressure. A gradient between the cavernous and brachial artery pressures of less than 35 mm Hg and equal pressure between the right and left cavernous arteries are normal.[25]

Cavernosometry and Cavernosography

Cavernosometry involves simultaneous saline infusion and intracorporeal pressure monitoring. A more physiologic refinement is the intracavernous injection of vasodilating agents such as papaverine + phentolamine, alprostadil, or a combination of the three drugs. The saline infusion rate necessary to maintain erection, and the drop in intracorporeal pressure 30 seconds after cessation of infusion, are thus directly related to the degree of venous leak. Gravity-infusion cavernosometry is a simpler and more economic alternative to the pump-infusion method.

Cavernosography involves the infusion of diluted radiocontrast solution into the corpora cavernosa during an artificial erection to visualize the site of venous leak. Cavernosometry and cavernosography always should be performed after activation of the veno-occlusive mechanism by intracavernous

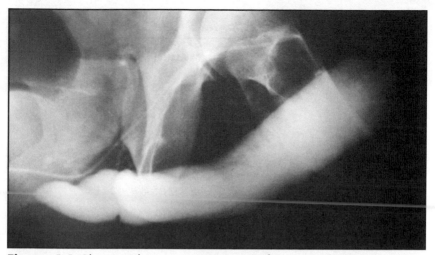

Figure 4-6: Pharmacologic cavernosogram of a man with normal veno-occlusive function. The radiocontrast material remains inside the corpora cavernosa, and the venous channels were not visualized.

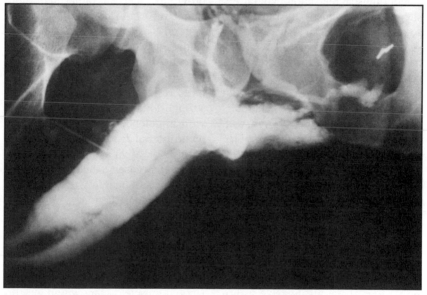

Figure 4-7: Large amount of venous leak through the crural, cavernous, and deep dorsal veins of the penis.

injection of vasodilators[26]; various leakage sites to the glans, corpus spongiosum, superficial and deep dorsal veins, and cavernous and crural veins can then be detected (Figures 4-6 and 4-7). Technical factors may influence the findings of cavernosometry and cavernosography. The study is done in a non-

Table 4-5: Smooth Muscle Content in the Corpora Cavernosa*

Patient Category	% Smooth Muscle (Corpora Cavernosa)
Potent (age)	
2-20	46.1
21-40	46.2
41-60	40.6
61-73	35.3
Old impotent	
with venous leak	19-36
with arterial insufficiency	10-25

*Wespes et al (1991, 1998)

sexual setting with little privacy, leading to patient anxiety and an adverse effect on erectile response. The phenomenon of incomplete trabecular smooth-muscle relaxation may falsely suggest veno-occlusive dysfunction in some normal subjects.[27] Therefore, repeated injections of vasodilators may be necessary to achieve complete smooth-muscle relaxation.[28] The normal maintenance rate in patients with complete smooth-muscle relaxation is reported to be less than 5 mL/min, with a pressure drop of less than 45 mm Hg from 150 mm Hg in 30 seconds after infusion is stopped.

Arteriography

Although angiography is likely the most accurate single test for evaluating the anatomy of the iliac, pudendal, and common penile arteries and their branches, its application has significant limitations. Like all invasive radiographic tests, the study is performed under artificial conditions, which may produce a significant sympathetic response and inhibit the erectile response. Inadequate vasodilation of the cavernous arteries, vasospasm induced by can-nulation, and injection of contrast solution may result in abnormal radiographic appearance.

Arteriography is most useful in providing anatomic rather than functional information. Because of the high cost and invasive nature of the study, only a small percentage of impotent patients are appropriate candidates (those who are candidates for arterial revascularization). Perhaps the strongest indication is in a young man with impotence secondary to a traumatic arterial disruption or in a patient with pelvic steal syndrome (rare). In these select cases, a detailed road map of the arterial anatomy is essential to surgical reconstruction.

Cavernous Assessment
Cavernous Smooth Muscle

Wespes et al observed an age-related and disease-dependent decrease in smooth-muscle content within the corpora cavernosa (Table 4-5).[29,30] The most severe lesions were observed in the erectile tissue, particularly in the smooth muscle of the trabeculae and helicine arteries, which had been reduced and replaced by connective tissue.

Nitric Oxide Synthase

Brock et al determined the presence of nitric oxide synthase (NOS) (as shown by nicotinamide adenine dinucleotide phosphate [NADP] diaphorase staining) in nerve fibers, smooth muscle, and sinusoid endothelium.[31] Abundant staining for NOS correlated significantly with a clinical history of cavernous nerve integrity.

Cavernous biopsy remains controversial. Proponents believe that it is essential for examining the cavernous tissue before arterial or venous surgery is contemplated. However, we believe that the less invasive tests, such as CIS and duplex ultrasonography, are adequate in predicting the integrity of the cavernous smooth muscle,[32] and more studies are needed before the routine use of cavernous biopsy can be recommended.

Conclusion

We have used the patient's goal-directed approach to impotence for the past 10 years. We recommend that every patient undergo a thorough medical and psychosexual history, a physical examination, and appropriate laboratory tests. Further diagnostic testing is tailored to the treatment option chosen by the patient. The physician should also consider the patient's age, general health, and concomitant medical disease and the goals and expectations of the patient and his partner in recommending tests and treatments.

References

1. Brenot PH: Male impotence— a historical perspective. *L'Esprit du Temps*, France, 1994.

2. Karacan I: Clinical value of nocturnal penile erection in the prognosis of impotence. *Med Aspects Hum Sex* 1970;4:27.

3. Bradley WE, Timm GW, Gallagher JM, et al: New method for continuous measurement of nocturnal penile tumescence and rigidity. *Urology* 1985;26:4-9.

4. Levine LA, Carroll RA: Nocturnal penile tumescence and rigidity in men without complaints of erectile dysfunction using a new quantitative analysis software. *J Urol* 1994;152:1103-1107.

5. Allen RP, Engel RM, Smolev JK, et al: Comparison of duplex ultrasonography and nocturnal penile tumescence in evaluation of impotence. *J Urol* 1994;151:1525-1529.

6. Hirshkowitz M, Ware JC: Studies of nocturnal penile tumescence and rigidity. In: Singer C, Weiner WJ, eds. *Sexual Dysfunction: A Neuro-Medical Approach.* Armonk, NY, Futura Publishing, 1994.

7. Kaplan HS: *The Evaluation of Sexual Disorders.* New York, Brunner/Mazel, 1983.

8. Hartmann U: Psychological evaluation and psychometry. In: Jonas U, Thon WF, Stief CG, eds. *Erectile Dysfunction.* Berlin, Springer-Verlag, 1991, pp 93-103.

9. Goldstein I, Krane RJ: Diagnosis and therapy of erectile dysfunction. In: Walsh PC, Retik AB, Stamey TA, et al, eds. *Campbell's Urology.* Philadelphia, WB Saunders, 1992.

10. Padma-Nathan H: Neurophysiological studies of sexual dysfunction. In: Singer C, Weiner WJ, eds. *Sexual Dysfunction: A Neuro-Medical Approach.* Armonk, NY, Futura Publishing, 1994, pp 101-115.

11. Gerstenberg TC, Bradley WE: Nerve conduction velocity measurement of dorsal nerve of penis in normal and impotent males. *Urology* 1983;21:90-92.

12. Abicht JH: Testing the autonomic system. In: Jonas U, Thon WF, Stief CG, eds. *Erectile Dysfunction.* Berlin, Springer-Verlag, 1991, pp 187-193.

13. Wagner G, Gerstenberg T, Levin RJ: Electrical activity of corpus cavernosum

during flaccidity and erection of the human penis: a new diagnostic method? *J Urol* 1989;142:723-725.

14. Stief CG, Djamilian M, Anton P, et al: Single potential analysis of cavernous electrical activity in impotent patients: a possible diagnostic method for autonomic cavernous dysfunction and cavernous smooth muscle degeneration. *J Urol* 1991;146:771-776.

15. Carter JN, Tyson JE, Tolis G, et al: Prolactin-screening tumors and hypogonadism in 22 men. *N Engl J Med* 1978; 299:847-852.

16. McClure RD, Marshall L: Endocrinologic sexual dysfunction. In: Singer C, Weiner WJ, eds. *Sexual Dysfunction: A Neuro-Medical Approach.* Armonk, NY, Futura Publishing, 1994, pp 245-273.

17. Metz P, Bengtsson J: Penile blood pressure. *Scand J Urol Nephrol* 1981; 15:161-164.

18. Virag R, Frydman D, Legman M, et al: Intracavernous injection of papaverine as a diagnostic and therapeutic method in erectile failure. *Angiology* 1984;35:79-87.

19. Abber JC, Lue TF, Orvis BR, et al: Diagnostic tests for impotence: a comparison of papaverine injection with the penile-brachial index and nocturnal penile tumescence monitoring. *J Urol* 1986;135: 923-925.

20. Lue TF, Tanagho EA: Physiology of erection and pharmacological management of impotence. *J Urol* 1987;137:829-836.

21. Pescatori ES, Hatzichristou DG, Namburi S, et al: A positive intracavernous injection test implies normal venoocclusive but not necessarily normal arterial function: a hemodynamic study. *J Urol* 1994;151:1209-1216.

22. Donatucci CF, Lue TF: The combined intracavernous injection and stimulation test: diagnostic accuracy. *J Urol* 1992;148:61-62.

23. Lue TF, Hricak H, Marich KW, et al: Vasculogenic impotence evaluated by high-resolution ultrasonography and pulsed Doppler spectrum analysis. *Radiology* 1985;155:777-781.

24. Benson CB, Vickers MA: Sexual impotence caused by vascular disease: diagnosis with duplex sonography. *AJR Am J Roentgenol* 1989;153:1149-1153.

25. Padma-Nathan H: Neurophysiological studies of sexual dysfunction. In: Singer C, Weiner WJ, eds. *Sexual Dysfunction: A Neuro-Medical Approach.* Armonk, NY, Futura Publishing, 1994, pp 101-115.

26. Lue TF, Hricak H, Schmidt RA, et al: Functional evaluation of penile veins by cavernosography in papaverine-induced erection. *J Urol* 1986;135:479-482.

27. Montague DK, Lakin MM: False diagnoses of venous leak impotence. *J Urol* 1992;148:148-149.

28. Hatzichristou DG, Saenz de Tejada I, Kupferman S, et al: In vivo assessment of trabecular smooth muscle tone, its application in pharmaco-cavernosometry and analysis of intracavernous pressure determinants. *J Urol* 1995;153:1126-1135.

29. Wespes E, Goes PM, Schiffmann S, et al: Computerized analysis of smooth muscle fibers in potent and impotent patients. *J Urol* 1991;146:1015-1017.

30. Wespes E, de Goes PM, Schulman CS: Age-related changes in the qualification of the intracavernous smooth muscles in potent men. *J Urol* 1998;159:99.

31. Brock G, Nunes L, Padma-Nathan H, et al: Nitric oxide synthase: a new diagnostic tool for neurogenic impotence. *Urology* 1993;42:412-417.

32. Persson C, Diederichs W, Lue TF, et al: Correlation of altered penile ultrastructure with clinical arterial evaluation. *J Urol* 1989;142:1462-1468.

Chapter 5

Psychosexual Counseling and Nonmedical Therapies

"Men with erectile dysfunction want to have a rigid penis. They and their partners are less interested in help with relationship and lifestyle issues. Fewer than 5% of erectile dysfunction patients attend further counseling."—Surridge et al[1]

Psychogenic erectile dysfunction is defined as the persistent inability to achieve and maintain erection for satisfactory sexual performance, caused predominantly or exclusively by psychological or interpersonal factors. In the Massachusetts Male Aging Study,[2] erectile dysfunction was significantly associated with depressive symptoms (odds ratio [OR]=2.88), pessimistic attitudes (OR=3.89), or a negative outlook on life (OR=2.30). In the National Health and Social Life Survey,[3] erectile dysfunction was reported to be significantly associated with emotional stress (OR=3.56) and a history of sexual coercion (OR=3.52).

Pathogenesis of Psychogenic Erectile Dysfunction

Psychosocial causes of sexual dysfunctions traditionally are divided into immediate and remote causes (Table 5-1).[4]

Bancroft[5] proposes that psychogenic arousal in men depends on a delicate balance between central excitatory and inhibitory mechanisms. While excessive inhibition may be associated with erectile or other sexual dysfunctions, insufficient inhibition alone could lead to development of high-risk sexual behaviors. Regarding the role of cognitive/attentional factors in psychogenic erectile dysfunction, studies suggest that it is not anxiety per se that is responsible for initiating or maintaining sexual arousal difficulties; rather, it is the alterations in perceptual and attentional processes that occur in sexually dysfunctional male and female patients.[6] Together, the molecular biology of psychogenic erectile dysfunction probably can be summarized as follows: instead of a full-throttle prosexual stimulation from the brain to the spinal erection center during a normal sexual act, the erection nerve of a patient with psychogenic erectile dysfunction receives only a lukewarm or distress signal, which impairs the release of neurotransmitters to the penis.

Diagnosis of Psychogenic Erectile Dysfunction

The diagnosis of psychogenic erectile dysfunction used to be made when an organic cause could not be found— a diagnosis of exclusion. With better

Table 5-1: Causes of Psychogenic Erectile Dysfunction

Immediate Causes

- Performance anxiety (fear of failure, adoption of spectator role)
- Lack of adequate stimulation, distracting stimuli
- Relationship conflicts: communication problems, lack of intimacy, power conflict, loss of sexual attraction, loss of trust

Early Developmental Causes

- Childhood sexual trauma
- Sexual identity problems
- Altered sexual orientation
- Unresolved parental attachments
- Religious or cultural taboos

understanding of the pathogenesis, psychogenic erectile dysfunction should be diagnosed only in the presence of specific and significant psychogenic factors (eg, performance anxiety, marital conflict). If necessary, a nocturnal penile tumescence and rigidity (NPTR) test can be performed to confirm the presence of normal neurovascular function.

Management of Psychogenic Erectile Dysfunction

As summarized by Rosen,[4] there are four categories of psychosocial therapies for erectile dysfunction: (1) anxiety reduction and desensitization, (2) cognitive-behavioral interventions, (3) increased sexual stimulation, and (4) interpersonal assertiveness and couples communication training. However, as found by the 1992 National Institutes of Health Consensus Conference on Erectile Dysfunction,[7] "Outcome data of psychological and behavioral

therapy have not been quantified, and evaluation of the success of specific techniques used in these treatments is poorly documented."

Based on many years of observation, Hengeveld[8] suggested contraindications for psychosexual therapy (Table 5-2); these may aid in the decision when referral to a psychologist is considered.

Anxiety Reduction and Desensitization

Masters and Johnson's[9] 'sensate focus' approach and Wolpe's[10] and Lazarus's[11] 'systematic desensitization' are methods used in overcoming performance anxiety and inhibitions typically associated with erectile dysfunction. Their aim was to detach sexuality from performance anxiety, inhibition, and guilt.

In the initial phase, the couple is advised to enjoy their bodies, using all senses in a relaxed and erotic way

Table 5-2: Contraindications to Psychosexual Therapy

Relative Contraindications to Psychosexual Therapy

- Uncooperative patient or sexual partner
- Low sex drive
- Homosexual orientation
- Psychosis or major mood disorder
- Major interpersonal problems with sexual partner
- Failure of previous psychosexual treatment

Relative Psychosexual Contraindications to Treatment (Injection, Implant)

- Unrealistic expectations
- Psychosis or major mood disorder
- Psychosomatic disorder (conversion disorder, chronic pain disorder, hypochondriasis)
- Substance abuse
- Crisis situation (divorce, grief, serious illness)
- Major interpersonal problem with sexual partner
- Sexual partner averse or psychiatrically disturbed

Modified from Hengeveld MW: Erectile disorder: a psychosexological review. In: Jonas U, Thon WF, Stief CG, eds. *Erectile Dysfunction*. Berlin, Springer-Verlag, 1991.

but to abstain completely from coitus. Subsequently, stimulation of sexual organs is encouraged, and when erection returns, the couple can then progress to coitus. Kaplan[12] emphasized the treatment of underlying personal or interpersonal conflicts. Others emphasize the importance of eliminating distorted beliefs, conflicts, and distractions and of enhancing the relationship.

Treatment Program

Sensate focus 1 involves learning how to sensually (not sexually) pleasure each other.[8] Caressing, stroking, and touching each other builds an affectionate bond between the partners and reduces sexual anxiety. The time, place, and room where this exercise is done should all be planned beforehand. The room should be warm, comfortable, and softly lit, and it should not be associated with any physical or emotional pressure. Avoid the bedroom if it has been the scene for many past sexual failures.

The couple should take a bath or shower to help them relax. Then they should go to the planned room, naked.

If the man has erectile dysfunction, he lies down on his back, with the woman using all of her senses to affect the man. However, she must avoid his genitals. The focus is to get used to different sensations. Nothing should be said in the early stages of therapy. After 15 minutes, the man turns over onto his stomach, and the woman continues. After 15 more minutes, the man and woman switch roles, with the woman lying down and the man touching her, avoiding her breasts and genitals. The couple should experiment with sensations that they are not familiar with. The process should take at least an hour, and once the couple is comfortable with this technique, they can use massage oil or talcum powder. At the end of the session, the couple should lie in each other's arms.

During therapy, the couple should discuss what they felt to give positive reinforcement to each other. When communication improves during therapy, the couple can continue to communicate during the exercises at home.

Sensate focus 2 involves the same technique as Sensate focus 1, except that the couple is allowed to look at each other's genitals but avoid stimulation. The idea is to give the couple a visual image of each other's genitals and to be comfortable with them as a part of sexual arousal.

Sensate focus (sexual) occurs when the couple is comfortable with the previous exercises. They can then begin gentle, light touching, in a teasing way. At this point, the couple begins to feel aroused. If the man is relaxed and having erections, the couple can move on to the next step.

Specific treatment is when the woman stimulates the man to erection and then stops, letting the erection subside. This is repeated twice more, allowing the man to concentrate on the sensations he receives while the woman stimulates him. This also builds his confidence that he is able to achieve and sustain an erection.

The next exercise involves the woman straddling the man, stimulating him to erection, and inserting his penis into her vagina. Then she does not move and allows the penis to become flaccid. She repeats this technique two more times. Once the couple is comfortable with this technique, the woman can begin to move around and stimulate the penis. Ejaculation should then occur, which achieves the goal, and the treatment program ends.

There are a few other exercises that may benefit the man. For a particularly tense and anxious patient, relaxation techniques may be useful. Other patients may benefit from a self-focus program. Self-focus programs help the patient to become more aware of his body and to determine what sensations he enjoys most. Finally, Kegel exercises can help the man and the woman.

Initially, Masters and Johnson[9] reported a 70% success rate in restoring erectile function. Subsequent reports placed the success rate in a range of 35% to 80% with a significant recurrence rate.[13,14] Psychosexual therapy is reported to be less successful in patients with primary erectile dysfunction.[15]

Cognitive-Behavioral Interventions

Cognitive restructuring techniques are used to overcome sexual ignorance and to challenge the unrealistic sexual expectations that typically accompany erectile dysfunction. Men (and their partners) frequently harbor gross misconceptions about the basic mechanisms and processes of erectile function and the causes of sexual dysfunction. The effects of illness and drugs, aging, and male-female differences in sexual response are additional common areas of ignorance. Self-hypnosis and fantasy training procedures have also been recommended for developing positive sexual imagery.[16,17]

This method of therapy aims at making couples more trusting and comfortable with sex. Often the focus is on lessening the fear of failure and directing attention to sensual and sexual pleasure. One approach replaces coitus with sexual learning exercises done at home. Cognitive-behavioral treatment works best when the physician takes the time to learn as much as possible about the patient and determines an individualized approach for every couple. A different strategy may need to be used for special cases. A patient who believes that his problem is physical and does not accept the fact that his problem may be psychological must be approached in a manner that resolves his psychological difficulties without him knowing it. The therapist may suggest that there is nothing detectably wrong with the patient's anatomy; however, stress may amplify erectile problems. The therapist could suggest to the patient to refrain from coitus but to continue to engage in sexual foreplay. By removing performance anxiety, the patient may achieve an erection and cure himself by disobeying the doctor.[8]

Banning intercourse is a technique that often helps patients. If a patient disobeys the physician's orders, he will have achieved a positive sexual experience that will help in creating more positive experiences in the future. If the patient disobeys the physician, but fails, the physician can just say that the patient tried intercourse too soon. Prohibiting intercourse is used because couples often focus too much on intercourse itself; instead the couple should concentrate on basics and relearn how to derive pleasure.

Education is important in this method of treatment. Couples must tell each other what arouses them. Sometimes, couples do not fully understand how to arouse their partners and basic arousal skills need to be taught. Generally, the more one partner learns about the other's body, the more they both learn how to give and receive sensual pleasure from each other. Sexual partners often develop routines that no longer work after several years. These couples need to communicate with each other and try new things to shift their foci from performance to pleasure.

Another technique involves expanding the patient's cognitive definition of sex. A patient may only associate specific concepts (such as love, happiness, and self-esteem) with sex, but by expanding the patient's thinking, sex may be significant in other parts of his life as well. Some men do not associate anything with sex until they enter the bed, and, as a result, they try to perform sexually with no 'warm-up'. By associating other concepts with sex, the mind is more in tune with sex, and the patient can build up to having sex.

Men often have self-destructive or interfering thoughts right before or during intercourse, such as, "I won't be able to please her... I will not be able to keep my erection." Therapists treat this by restructuring the man's thinking. The man would ideally begin to think in a way that focuses more on sensual pleasure rather than performance. By redefining what the patient believes is sex, the patient also learns to enjoy the sensual aspects of sex.

Some couples have trouble communicating about sex. Others are limited in their sexual behavior. These couples may find erotic material helpful in broadening the basis of their sexual relationships. Books or videos may provide examples of techniques that the couple was too shy to discuss before.

Enhancing Sexual Stimulation

It has frequently been observed that erectile dysfunction is most sexually debilitating for couples with limited sexual repertoires and few alternatives to intercourse.[18] For these individuals, the male's inability to achieve a firm and lasting erection typically results in a complete cessation of all sexual activity. In one early study, sexual communication training was found to be superior to sensate focus alone in the treatment of secondary erectile dysfunction.[19]

LoPiccolo[20] has emphasized the critical role of the female partner's attitude toward nonintercourse forms of sexual stimulation. If the patient can be reassured that his partner finds their lovemaking highly pleasurable and that she is sexually fulfilled by the orgasms he gives her through manual and oral stimulation, his performance anxiety will be greatly reduced. From this perspective, treatment is often focused on the sexual receptivity of the partner to nonintercourse forms of stimulation.

Among older men, in particular, there is an increasing need for direct, tactile stimulation of the penis, along with a decreasing responsiveness to psychogenic forms of stimulation.[21] Thus, the older male may require extended manual or oral stimulation of the penis to achieve adequate erection for intercourse.

Interpersonal (Couple) Therapies

Interpersonal and couples issues play a major role in many, if not most, cases of erectile dysfunction. Relationship conflicts may be a primary source of the sexual difficulty or may serve to exacerbate or maintain the male's inability to achieve adequate erections. Among the specific areas of intervention, Rosen et al[22] have identified three major dimensions of couples conflict that are important to consider. These are (1) status and dominance issues, (2) intimacy and trust, and (3) loss of sexual attraction.

Several therapies also have been proposed for single males with chronic erectile dysfunction.[23,24] Treatment strategies include sexual attitude change, assertiveness training, masturbation exercises, and social skills development. Previously, sexual surrogate therapy had been used in several centers for treatment of single males.[25,26] Despite the value of this approach in some cases, the potential risks and uncertain legal status of surrogate therapy have greatly limited its use.

Psychoanalytic Individual Therapy

This therapy is based on the theory that the sexual dysfunction represents an underlying subconscious conflict, and psychoanalytical principles are used to treat the neurosis that has developed from the conflict. This method involves a classical approach in which the patient learns a new way of seeing himself. If a patient's erectile problems are associated with some sort of emotional response that no longer applies to him, he can learn to create a new image of himself that will break through certain emotional barriers and cure his erectile problems. This type of treatment has a drawback in that it requires prolonged, intense therapy. There have not been any data showing the success of this kind of therapy.

Lifestyle Changes

Although it is difficult to prove its beneficial effect, a change of lifestyle should be encouraged (regular exercise, a healthy diet, smoking cessation, alcohol in moderation only). In rabbit experiments, the deleterious effect of a high-cholesterol diet on the cavernous smooth muscle was reversed several weeks after cholesterol was removed from the diet.[27] We found that the best time to discuss this with the patient is during vascular evaluation. If the patient is made aware that penile vascular disease is part of a generalized vascular disease that may involve other organs, he will more likely accept the advice.

Long-distance bicycle riding is another risk factor that should be discussed. Changing the bicycle seat or pursuing another form of exercise may be necessary if penile vascular compromise is found.

Pelvic Floor Muscle Exercise

Claes et al[28] studied the anatomy of the ischiocavernosus muscle in cadavers and suggested that it influences venous drainage of the corpus cavernosum. They gave 155 patients intensive physiotherapy consisting of electrical stimulation of the ischiocavernosus muscle, graded pelvic floor exercises with muscle training, and a home exercise program for lying, sitting, and standing positions. Intensive practice of increasing duration was encouraged. After 4 months, 69 patients were cured, and 42 patients had improved.

References

1. Surridge DH, Lee JC, Morales A, et al: Penile rigidity may supersede partner and counseling issues. *J Urol* 1998;159:29.

2. Feldman HA, Goldstein I, Hatzichrisou DG, et al: Impotence and its medical and psychosocial correlates: results of the Massachusetts Male Aging Study. *J Urol* 1994; 151:54-61.

3. Lauman EO, Paik A, Rosen RC: Sexual dysfunction in the United States: prevalence and predictors. *JAMA* 1999;281:537-544.

4. Rosen RC: Psychogenic erectile dysfunction. Classification and management. *Urol Clin North Am* 2001;28:269-278.

5. Bancroft J: Central inhibition of sexual response in the male: a theoretical perspective. *Neurosci Biobehav Rev* 1999; 23:763-784.

6. Cohen AS, Rosen RC, Goldstein L: EEG hemispheric asymmetry during sexual arousal: psychophysiological patterns in responsive, unresponsive, and dysfunctional men. *J Abnorm Psychol* 1985;94:580-590.

7. Consensus development conference statement. National Institutes of Health. Impotence. December 7-9, 1992. *Int J Impot Res* 1993;5:181-284.

8. Hengeveld MW: Erectile disorder: a psychosexological review. In: Jones U, Thon WF, Stief CG, eds. *Erectile Dysfunction*. Berlin, Springer-Verlag, 1991.

9. Masters WH, Johnson VE: *Human Sexual Inadequacy*. Boston, Little Brown, 1970.

10. Wolpe J: *Psychotherapy by Reciprocal Inhibition*. Stanford, CA, Stanford University Press, 1958.

11. Lazarus AA: The treatment of a sexually inadequate man. In: Ullmann LP, Drasner L, eds. *Case Studies in Behavior Modification*. New York, Holt, Rinehart and Winston, 1965, pp 243-260.

12. Kaplan HS: *The New Sex Therapy*. New York, Brunner/Mazel, 1974.

13. LoPiccolo J, Stock WE: Treatment of sexual dysfunction. *J Consult Clin Psychol* 1986;54:158-167.

14. Hengeveld MW: Erectile dysfunction: a sexological and psychiatric review. *World J Urol* 1983;1:227.

15. Vickers MA Jr, De Nobrega AM, Dluhy RG: Diagnosis and treatment of psychogenic erectile dysfunction in a urological setting: outcomes of 18 consecutive patients. *J Urol* 1993;149:1258-1261.

16. Araoz DL: Hypnosex therapy. *J Clin Hypn* 1983;26:37-41.

17. Brown JM, Chaves JF: Hypnosis in the treatment of sexual dysfunction. *J Sex Marital Ther* 1980;6:63-74.

18. Leiblum SR, Rosen RC. Couples therapy for erectile disorders: conceptual and clinical considerations. *J Sex Marital Ther* 1991;17:147-159.

19. Takefman J, Brender W: An analysis of the effectiveness of two components in the treatment of erectile dysfunction. *Arch Sex Behav* 1984;13:321-340.

20. LoPiccolo J: Postmodern sex therapy for erectile failure. In: Rosen RC, Leiblum SR, eds. *Erectile Disorders: Assessment and Treatment*. New York, Guilford Press, 1992, pp 171-197.

21. Segraves RT, Segraves KB: Aging and drug effects on male sexuality. In: Rosen RC, Leiblum SR, eds. *Erectile Disorders: Assessment and Treatment*. New York, Guilford Press, 1992, pp 96-140.

22. Rosen RC, Leiblum SR, Spector IP: Psychologically based treatment for male erectile disorder: a cognitive-interpersonal model. *J Sex Marital Ther* 1994;20:67-85.

23. Reynolds B: Psychological treatment of erectile dysfunction in men without partners: outcome results and a new direction. *J Sex Marital Ther* 1991;17:136-146.

24. Stravynski A, Greenberg D: The treatment of sexual dysfunction in single men. *J Sex Marital Ther* 1990;15.

25. Apfelbaum B: The ego-analytic approach to individual body-work sex therapy: Five case examples. *J Sex Res* 1984;20:44-70.

26. Dauw DC: Evaluating the effectiveness of the SECS surrogate-assisted sex therapy model. *J Sex Res* 1988;24:269-275.

27. Kim JH, Klyachkin ML, Svendsen E, et al: Experimental hypercholesterolemia in rabbits induces cavernosal atherosclerosis with endothelial and smooth muscle cell dysfunction. *J Urol* 1994;151:198-205.

28. Claes H, van Hove J, van de Voorde W, et al: Pelvi-perineal rehabilitation for dysfunctioning erections. A clinical and anatomo-physiologic study. *Int J Impot Res* 1993;5:13-26.

Chapter 6

Hormonal Therapy

I refer patients with thyroid, adrenal, pituitary, or hypothalamic dysfunction to endocrinologists for further work-up and treatment. This chapter, therefore, is limited to hypogonadism and hyperprolactinemia.

Hypogonadism

In young hypogonadal men, testosterone replacement is clearly the treatment of choice. However, in older patients, the risks (Table 6-1) may outweigh the benefits because testosterone may speed the growth of a hyperplastic prostate or occult prostate cancer. Nevertheless, in a number of older hypogonadal patients, libido and erectile function can be restored by testosterone therapy. This option should not be denied to these patients. When a patient desires this therapy, we routinely perform a digital rectal examination and obtain a serum prostate-specific antigen (PSA) level. When in doubt, ultrasound-guided biopsy also is done before androgen therapy is given. Patients are followed every 6 months with a rectal examination and serum PSA as long as they are on therapy.

The common androgen preparations are modifications by esterification of the 17-β-hydroxyl group or alkylation at the 17-α group (Table 6-2).[1] The alkylated testosterone preparations can be given orally, but absorption may be erratic, and these preparations may carry a risk of hepatotoxicity (eg, cholestasis, hepatitis, benign, and malignant tumors). The esterified preparation makes the testosterone more soluble in the fatty vehicles used for parenteral injection and slow release. The long-acting forms, testosterone cypionate (Virilon®) and enanthate (Delatestryl®), are the drugs of choice for replacement therapy. In a study by Sokol et al, hypogonadal men receiving 200 mg of testosterone enanthate demonstrated a peak (supraphysiologic) level at 24 hours, which fell below eugonadal levels by day 9.[2] Therefore, the recommended dosage is 200 mg IM every 2 to 3 weeks. If the patient complains of decreased libido and energy a few days before the next injection, testosterone level should be checked and dose interval should be shortened if the level is low. Some patients with hypogonadotropic hypogonadism may respond better to gonadotropin-releasing hormone or clomiphene (Clomid®) 50 mg/d.

Transdermal Testosterone Replacement

Two transdermal patches, Testoderm® and Androderm®, are approved

Table 6-1: Potential Benefits and Side Effects of Testosterone Therapy

Benefits	Side Effects
• Prevents osteoporosis	• Polycythemia and venous thrombosis
• Increases muscle mass and strength	• Prostate growth and urinary retention
• Increases energy	• Increased prostate-specific antigen (PSA)
• Increases libido	• Potential growth of prostate cancer
• Better erection (10%-20% only)	• Liver toxicity (oral preparation)
	• Skin allergy (dermal patch)

by the Food and Drug Administration. The former is applied to the scrotal area and the latter to any skin surface. In clinical trials, the transdermal system increased serum testosterone concentrations to within normal in more than 90% of patients. The most common adverse events are dermal: itching (7%), chronic skin irritation (2% to 5%), and allergic contact dermatitis (4%). In patients on long-term therapy, periodic checks of hematocrit (to detect polycythemia), liver function, and PSA levels are recommended. The initial recommended dose of Androderm® is one system applied nightly for 24 hours, which provides about 5 mg/d of testosterone. Skin irritation is a troublesome side effect in many patients. Pretreatment with triamcinolone acetonide 0.1% cream has been shown to reduce the severity and incidence of persistent, bothersome skin irritation.[3] The initial therapeutic dose of Testoderm® is 6 mg/d applied daily to the shaved scrotal skin. A Testoderm® transdermal system (TTS) that delivers 5 mg/d of testosterone can be applied to any preferred skin site without the need for rotation. In clinical studies, the most common adverse effects were transient itching (12%), moderate to severe erythema (3%), and headache (5%). Another delivery method is testosterone 1% gel (Andro-Gel®) transdermal preparation. It is recommended to start with 5 g/every morning and adjust the amount according to the blood testosterone level. Morning serum testosterone level may be measured for titration of proper dose. These preparations are Schedule III controlled substances under the Anabolic Steroids Control Act.

Although endocrinopathy can certainly contribute to impotence, its role may result from its effects on central mechanisms (libido) rather than on the penile tissue itself; its overall contribution as a directly treatable cause of impotence is unclear. The efficacy of hormonal replacement in hypogonadal impotence also has been rather disappointing. Morales et al reported only a 9% response rate for patients treated with oral androgen replacement.[4] Most older patients more likely suffer from concomitant neurovascular

Table 6-2: Androgen Preparations[1]

Preparation	Dose (mg)	Route	Schedule
17-alkylated androgens			
Methyltestosterone (Android®)	25-50	sublingual	daily
Fluoxymesterone (Halotestin®)	5-10	oral	daily
Transdermal			
Testoderm®	4-6	scrotal skin	daily
Testoderm® TTS	5	skin	daily
Androderm®	5	skin	daily
Esterified testosterone			
Propionate	50	IM	3x/week
Cypionate (Virilon®)	200	IM	every 2-3 weeks
Enanthate (Delatestryl®)	200	IM	every 2-3 weeks

insufficiency than from androgen deficiency alone. If the aim of androgen replacement therapy is to restore erectile function, testosterone is a relatively poor choice.

Hyperprolactinemia

In patients with hyperprolactinemia with or without hypogonadism, testosterone therapy does not improve sexual function. Treatment should first be aimed at eliminating the offending drugs, such as estrogens, morphine, sedatives, or neuroleptics. Bromocriptine (Parlodel®) is a dopamine agonist that lowers the prolactin level and restores testosterone to normal. It is used to reduce tumor size in patients with a prolactin-secreting tumor. The initial dose is one half to one 2.5-mg tablet daily. An additional tablet can be added as tolerated every 3 to 7 days until an optimal therapeutic response is achieved. The therapeutic dosage is usually 5 mg to 7.5 mg and ranges from 2.5 to 15 mg/d. Surgery occasionally may be needed if the response is not satisfactory. In a study of 600 randomly selected patients, Netto and Claro reported that moderate elevations of prolactin levels, without any associated disorder, occurred in 3.8% (23/600) of patients.[5] In patients with prolactin levels ranging from 20 to 40 ng/mL, bromocriptine brought the values down to normal in all, but only one patient achieved full erection. In patients with levels higher than 40 ng/mL, 9 of 11 achieved normal levels after treatment, and 77.7% achieved full erection. These findings indicate that, in patients with a mild prolactin elevation, other factors such as vascular or neurologic deficit may be the underlying cause of erectile dysfunction. The treatment of choice for pituitary adenoma (usually in patients with marked prolactin elevation) is bromocriptine or surgical ablation.

Male Menopause

Male menopause (andropause), if it exists, is a gradual decline of hormone levels and body function, and is different from female menopause. Symptoms of andropause may include hot flashes, mood swings, insomnia, depression, irritability, decreased libido, impotence, weakness, lethargy, loss of lean body mass, and decreased bone mass. The relationship of these symptoms to declining androgen levels is controversial, and the benefit of androgen therapy remains unproven. Testosterone, dehydroepiandrosterone (DHEA), and growth hormone have been touted as a 'fountain of youth,' without the mention of possible adverse effects. Until more scientific studies prove its beneficial effect in reversing aging, testosterone should be reserved for those with genuine hypogonadism.

References

1.   McClure RD, Marshall L: Endocrinologic sexual dysfunction. In: Singer C, Weiner WJ, eds. *Sexual Dysfunction: A Neuro-Medical Approach*. Armonk, NY, Futura Publishing, 1994, p 245.

2.   Sokol RZ, Palacios A, Campfield LA, et al: Comparison of the kinetics of injectable testosterone in eugonadal and hypogonadal men. *Fertil Steril* 1982; 37:425-430.

3.   Wilson DE, Kaidbey K, Boike CS, et al: Use of topical corticosteroid cream in the pretreatment of skin reactions associated with Androderm® Testosterone Transdermal System. In: Program and abstracts of the 7th annual meeting of the Endocrine Society. Abstract pp 1-323, Minneapolis, June 1997.

4.   Morales A, Johnston B, Heaton JW, et al: Oral androgens in the treatment of hypogonadal impotent men. *J Urol* 1994; 152:1115-1118.

5.   Netto NR Jr, Claro J de A: The importance of hyperprolactinemia in impotence. *Rev Paul Med* 1993;111:454-455.

Chapter 7

Pharmacotherapy: Oral and Topical Agents

"The desire to take medicine is perhaps the greatest feature that distinguishes men from animals."—Sir William Osler

Medication Change

When a patient complains of sexual dysfunction after taking a particular medication, the clinician must determine whether the problem is related to loss of sexual drive, impaired erection, or difficult ejaculation. In many situations, changing the medication to one belonging to a different class of agents may be helpful. For example, older antihypertensive drugs such as methyldopa (Aldomet®) and reserpine have a high incidence of sexual dysfunction because of their central effect; substitution with newer drugs, such as calcium channel blockers or angiotensin-converting enzyme (ACE) inhibitors, may reverse the dysfunction in some patients. Patients who complain of sexual dysfunction after taking antidepressants may also benefit from substitution with trazodone (Desyrel®) or bupropion (Wellbutrin®), which are known to improve erectile function in some patients. If medication change does not improve sexual function, then vascular, neurologic, or hormonal causes are more likely, and an appropriate work-up should be conducted.

Centrally Acting Drugs

Adrenergic, dopaminergic, and serotonergic receptors occupy the brain centers associated with libido, penile erection, and ejaculation. Therefore, a number of drugs stimulate sexual function, presumably through their action on these receptors.

Adrenoceptor antagonists. In studies of human corpus cavernosum erectile tissue, Traish et al[1,2] reported the presence of α_1 A, B, and D and α_2 A, B, and C adrenoceptor subtypes. Other functional studies suggest that α_1-adrenoceptors predominate in the human cavernous tissue and that α_2-adrenoceptors prevail in the cavernous artery.[3,4] The addition of an α-blocker, doxazosin (Cardura®), was recently shown to have a beneficial effect in patients with erectile dysfunction for whom intracavernosal alprostadil (prostaglandin E_1 [PGE_1]) therapy alone fails. The synergistic effects of vascular dilation and blockade of sympathetic inhibition may explain this response.[5]

Phentolamine is an α_1- and α_2-adrenoceptor blocker that has been used in combination with papaverine for intracavernous injection. Oral phentolamine (Vasomax®) has been reported to improve erectile function in some patients.[6,7] The results of two clinical trials are shown in Table 7-1.

Yohimbine (Yocon®, Yohimex™, Aphrodyne®), an α_2-adrenergic an-

Table 7-1: Effect of Oral Phentolamine (Vasomax®) on Patients With Minimal Erectile Dysfunction in Two Clinical Trials

Study 1

	Placebo	40 mg	80 mg
Number of patients	148	152	159
% responders*	16	37	45

Study 2

	Placebo	40 mg
Number of patients	145	148
% responders*	21	34

Side effects: headache, facial flushing, nasal congestion

* A responder is any patient whose end point International Index of Erectile Function domain score improved by at least one clinical dysfunction class and who met at least the criteria for mild to moderate dysfunction at end point.

tagonist, is obtained from the bark of the yohimbe tree. In a controlled randomized study of patients with organic erectile dysfunction receiving 6 mg of yohimbine orally three times a day for 10 weeks, no statistically significant difference was found from those taking placebo.[8] However, in a study of patients with psychogenic erectile dysfunction, a positive response rate of 62% was found, while the placebo group only achieved a 16% response rate.[9]

Dopaminergic agonist. Apomorphine is a D_1 and D_2 dopaminergic receptor agonist known to cause yawning and erection in animals and humans. Lal et al demonstrated that it induces erection when injected subcutaneously.[10] A sublingual formulation of apomorphine (Uprima®) is being marketed in Europe for the treatment of erectile dysfunction. In a randomized, double-blind, crossover study of 296 heterosexual men with erectile dysfunction of various etiologies and severities,[11] the intercourse rate from 3 mg sublingual apomorphine (48%) was higher than that from placebo (34%, $P < 0.001$). Median time to erection was 18.8 min.

The 3-mg dose was not significantly different from a 4-mg dose in the evaluation of efficacy variables, but the incidence of adverse events was higher with 4 mg. Nausea was the most common event, reported by 3.3% of patients on 3 mg vs 14.1% on 4 mg; in the placebo comparison, nausea was reported by 7% of patients taking 3 mg sublingual apomorphine vs 1.1% of those taking placebo. Vasovagal syncope episodes were reported in <1% of patients. Other reported side effects are summarized in Table 7-2. Uprima® is not available in the United States.[12]

Table 7-2: Side Effects of Sublingual Apomorphine

Dose	2 mg	3 mg	4 mg
Patients (number)	849	804	747
Any symptoms	11.2%	13.4%	18.3%
Nausea	3.2%	4.7%	7.2%
Dizziness	2.0%	1.6%	3.2%
Headache	2.2%	3.6%	2.9%
Vasodilation	0.9%	0.9%	1.9%
Sweating	0.2%	1.0%	1.9%

Serotonergic drugs. Trazodone is a mild antidepressant with a rare incidence of priapism. Its effect on penile erection is thought to result from serotonergic and α-adrenolytic activity. Trazodone has been shown to enhance nocturnal erections.[13] The combination of trazodone and yohimbine also has been reported to improve erectile function in some patients.[14] The main problem of trazodone is its sedative effect, which may render sexual activity more difficult. Some patients learn to take advantage of better nocturnal erections with trazodone and engage in sexual activity in the morning when the sedative effect is no longer a problem.

Peripherally Acting Drugs

Some oral vasoactive drugs improve erectile function. In a double-blind, randomized clinical trial by Korenman and Viosca,[15] patients were given 12 weeks of treatment with placebo or 400 mg t.i.d. of pentoxifylline (Trental®). Therapy increased the penile brachial pressure index, and a significant number of men reported improved erectile function.

Phosphodiesterase Type 5 Inhibitors

Phosphodiesterase type 5 (PDE 5) inhibitors prolong the relaxant effect of cyclic guanosine monophosphate (cGMP) in penile smooth muscle. During sexual stimulation, nitric oxide (NO) is released into the penile smooth muscle from nonadrenergic/noncholinergic (NANC) neurons. NO activates guanylyl cyclase, leading to increased levels of cGMP, which then relaxes cavernous smooth muscle and produces penile erection. When the breakdown of cGMP is blocked by PDE 5 inhibitors, the concentration of cGMP increases, and its relaxant effects on penile smooth muscle are prolonged (Figure 7-1). Importantly, PDE 5 inhibitors have no effect on erection in the absence of sexual stimulation when NO and cGMP are at minimal basal levels.

Sildenafil

Since its introduction in March 1998, sildenafil citrate (Viagra®) has drastically changed the management of erectile dysfunction (Figure 7-2). Sildenafil treatment has been evalu-

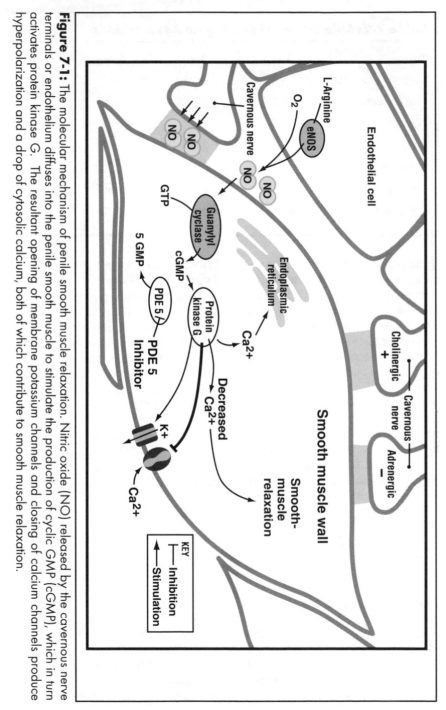

Figure 7-1: The molecular mechanism of penile smooth muscle relaxation. Nitric oxide (NO) released by the cavernous nerve terminals or endothelium diffuses into the penile smooth muscle to stimulate the production of cyclic GMP (cGMP), which in turn activates protein kinase G. The resultant opening of membrane potassium channels and closing of calcium channels produce hyperpolarization and a drop of cytosolic calcium, both of which contribute to smooth muscle relaxation.

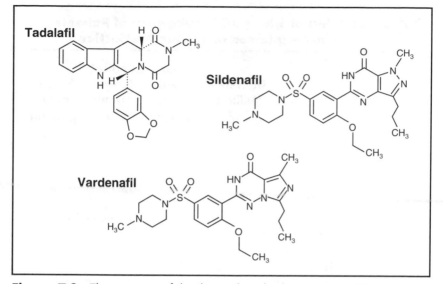

Figure 7-2: The structure of the three phosphodiesterase 5 inhibitors available in the United States.

ated in more than 90 placebo-controlled and open-label clinical trials encompassing more than 8,000 patients. Clinical response is dose dependent, with 63% of patients who took a 25-mg dose reporting improved erection and 82% reporting improvement with a 100-mg dose.[16] The number of erections and penile rigidity were improved,[17] as was overall satisfaction with treatment and orgasmic function. Rates of successful intercourse averaged 1.3 per week with 50 to 100 mg of sildenafil, compared to 0.4 in the placebo group. However, the trials have found that sildenafil has no effect on sexual drive. The effect on subgroups of patients is shown in Table 7-3.[18] In my clinical experience, sildenafil seems to work well in patients with psychogenic or mild to moderate neurovascular insufficiency. It is less effective in patients with venous leak or cavernous nerve injury (eg, within 6 months of radical prostatectomy).

Clinical safety data pooled from more than 3,700 patients with more than 1,600 years of medication exposure have shown that most adverse events from sildenafil are mild to moderate and self-limited.[19] Common complaints include headache (16%), flushing (10%), dyspepsia (7%), nasal congestion (4%), and abnormal vision (3%) described as a mild and transient blue tinge or increased sensitivity to light. This is caused by the effect of sildenafil on PDE 6, an enzyme found in the retina. (Sildenafil is about 10-fold as potent for PDE 5 as for PDE 6.) The incidence of adverse effects increases with larger doses. At 100-mg doses, dyspepsia occurred in 17% of patients and abnormal vision in 11%. The discontinuation rate from all adverse events was similar for sildenafil and placebo groups, 2.5% and 2.3%, respectively.

Table 7-3: Effect of Sildenafil in Subgroups of Patients Who Complained of Erectile Dysfunction

		Diabetes Mellitus (n=268)	Spinal Cord Injury (n=178)	Radical Prosta-tectomy (n=91)	Psycho-genic (n=179)
Successful intercourse	Placebo	12%	13%	—	29%
	Sildenafil*	48%	59%	72% (BN), 50% (UN), 15% (NN)	70%

n = number of patients; BN = bilateral nerve sparing; UN = unilateral nerve sparing; NN = non-nerve sparing

*Sildenafil dose: 50-100 mg

Source: Sildenafil package insert and Zippe et al[18]

Table 7-4: Recommendations for Sildenafil and the Cardiac Patient[20]

Contraindicated in:

- Patients taking long-acting or short-acting nitrate drugs

Caution should be exercised in:

- Patients with stable coronary disease (pre-sildenafil treadmill test may be indicated to assess the risk of cardiac ischemia during sexual intercourse)

- Patients with congestive heart failure who have borderline low blood pressure and low volume status

- Patients who are on a complicated, multidrug, antihypertension therapy regimen

- Patients who are on other medications or have conditions that can prolong the duration of action of sildenafil

---

Adverse cardiovascular events were mild and transient in most cases and were similar for sildenafil and placebo groups. The rate of serious cardiovascular events such as myocardial infarctions was similar at 1.7 and 1.4 events (per 1,000 man-years of treatment) for the sildenafil and placebo groups, respectively.[19] A word of caution is warranted, however, because studies excluded patients using nitrates and patients with significant concomitant medical conditions. Most of the 130 sildenafil-related deaths re-

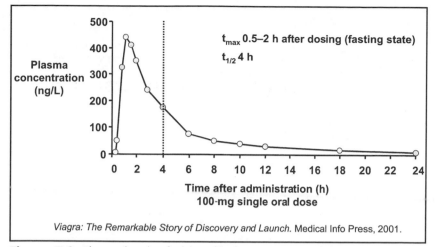

Figure 7-3: Plasma levels of sildenafil after 100-mg oral dose.

ported to the Food and Drug Administration (FDA) between March and November 1998 were associated with patients who had underlying cardiovascular disease. Therefore, the clinician must carefully assess the patient's cardiovascular status before prescribing sildenafil. In response to the concerns of physicians and the public, the American Heart Association has published recommendations for assessing patients before starting sildenafil therapy (Table 7-4).[20]

Sildenafil is absorbed well in the fasting state, reaching maximal plasma concentrations within 30 to 120 minutes (mean 60 minutes, Figure 7-3). The recommended starting dose is 50 mg, taken 1 hour before sexual activity. Depending on effectiveness and side effects, the dose can be increased to 100 mg or decreased to 25 mg. The maximum recommended frequency is once a day. Sildenafil is mainly metabolized by the liver. A lower starting dose of 25 mg should be used in patients more

than 65 years of age, in those with hepatic or renal impairment, and in those on concomitant use of P-450 3A4 inhibitors (eg, erythromycin, ketoconazole, itraconazole). Patients taking nitrates should not be given sildenafil because hypotension and cardiac compromise may result.

Some clinicians have suggested that sildenafil can improve clitoral blood flow and genital arousal in women; however, data supporting this application are lacking. Thus, use of sildenafil in women should not be encouraged until placebo-controlled, double-blind trials prove its effectiveness.

Recent concerns about cost and health-care reimbursement have also emerged. In an environment of competitive managed care, the use of sildenafil as a medical necessity is carefully scrutinized in many countries. Practicing in an era of limited resources, the treating physician should prescribe sildenafil only to those patients who would benefit most from it.

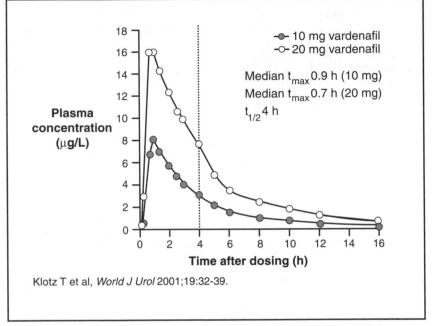

Figure 7-4: Plasma levels of vardenafil after 10- and 20-mg oral dose.

Vardenafil

Vardenafil hydrochloride (Levitra®) is the generic name for a new and more potent PDE 5 inhibitor (Figure 7-2).[21-23] In studies that compare vardenafil with sildenafil under the same conditions, vardenafil was nine times more potent than sildenafil and twofold to fourfold more specific for PDE 5 than for PDE 6 and PDE 1 than sildenafil.[24] Vardenafil reached its highest concentration in the blood after 35 to 50 minutes.[25-27] Repeated administration of 40-mg doses did not seem to cause significant accumulation in the blood.[28] Its half-life is 4 to 5 hours (Figure 7-4).[25,26] The pharmacokinetic data suggest that vardenafil is rapidly eliminated, and, therefore, any adverse events will be of short duration. A RigiScan® study after 20 mg of var-denafil showed that the erection time (>60% rigidity) was doubled compared with placebo.[26,28]

In a phase II study of 600 patients randomized to take 5 mg, 10 mg, or 20 mg vardenafil or placebo, 80% of patients on 20 mg vardenafil reported improved erections compared with 30% on placebo (Figure 7-5).[29] Patients' diaries showed that those taking vardenafil had a statistically improved rate of completed attempts (>70%) for all three doses compared with placebo (40%). When efficacy was analyzed over time, other measures of sexual function—such as orgasmic function, intercourse satisfaction, and overall satisfaction—significantly improved during the first 4 weeks. Improvement was maintained over the course of the 12-week study period

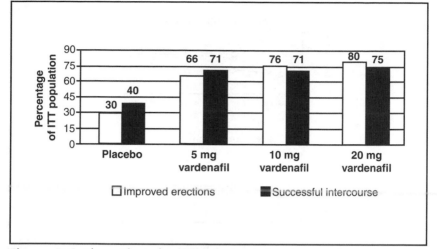

Figure 7-5: Phase IIb study: general population. Improved erections were measured by the percentage of the intent-to-treat (ITT) population replying yes to the global assessment question, "Has the treatment you have been taking over the past 4 weeks improved your erection?" after 12 weeks of vardenafil or placebo treatment. Total n for each group: 134 for placebo, 140 for 5 mg, 129 for 10 mg, and 138 for 20 mg. Successful intercourse was derived from ITT patient diaries where a successful attempt was defined by attempting, penetrating, and completing intercourse with ejaculation after 12 weeks of vardenafil or placebo treatment.
Adapted from Porst H et al, *Int J Impot Res* 2001;13:192-199.

Table 7-5: Incidence of Any Adverse Event in Phase II Study

% Adverse Events	Placebo n=152	Vardenafil 5 mg n=147	Vardenafil 10 mg n=141	Vardenafil 20 mg n=150
Headache	3.9%	6.8%	8.5%	15.3%
Flushing	0.7%	10.2%	11.3%	11.3%
Dyspepsia	0%	0.7%	2.8%	6.7%
Rhinitis	3.35%	4.8%	2.8%	7.3%
Visual*	0.7%	0%	0.7%	2.8%

*No blue color vision reported

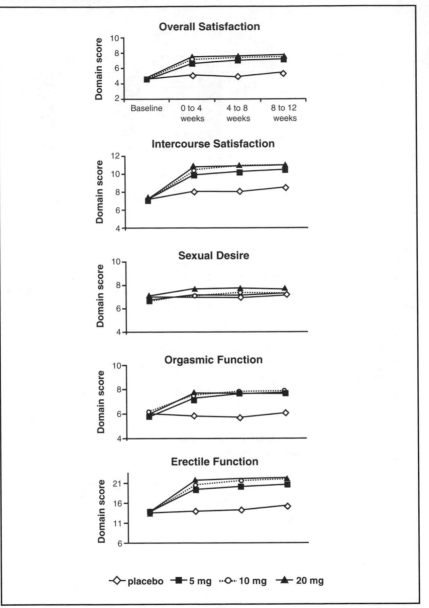

Figure 7-6: The International Index of Erectile Function (IIEF) scores in patients taking placebo or 5, 10, or 20 mg of vardenafil during a 12-week trial. Adapted from Young J, Auerbach S, Porst H, et al: Vardenafil (a new selective PDE 5 inhibitor) significantly improved all IIEF domains in patients with erectile dysfunction and showed a favorable safety profile: results at 4 and 12 weeks of treatment. Poster presentation at the American Urological Association, 2001.

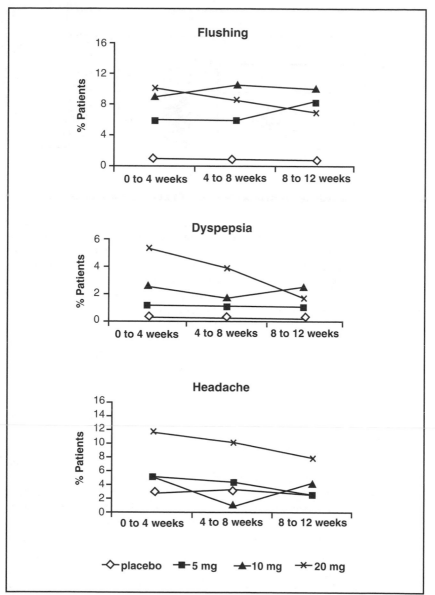

Figure 7-7: The percentage of patients who complained of dyspepsia or headache decreases with time during the 12-week vardenafil trial. Complaints of flushing do not decrease. Adapted from Young J, Auerbach S, Porst H, et al: Vardenafil (a new selective PDE 5 inhibitor) significantly improved all IIEF domains in patients with erectile dysfunction and showed a favorable safety profile: results at 4 and 12 weeks of treatment. Poster presentation at the American Urological Association, 2001.

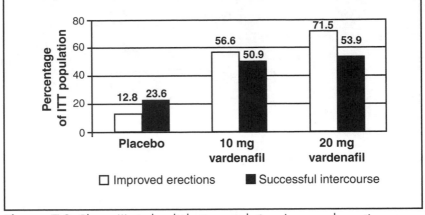

Figure 7-8: Phase III study: diabetic population. Improved erections were measured by the percentage of the intent-to-treat (ITT) population replying yes to the global assessment question, "Has the treatment you have been taking over the past 4 weeks improved your erection?" after 12 weeks of vardenafil or placebo treatment. Total n for each group: 133 for placebo, 137 for 10 mg, and 131 for 20 mg. Successful intercourse was derived from ITT patient diaries after 12 weeks of vardenafil or placebo treatment.
Adapted from Goldstein I, Young J, Fischer J, et al: Vardenafil, a new highly selective PDE 5 inhibitor, improves erectile function in patients with diabetes mellitus. Poster presentation at the American Diabetes Association, 2001.

(Figure 7-6).[30] Analysis of subsets of patients revealed that vardenafil improved erection in young and old men, in men with mild to severe erectile dysfunction, and in men with organic, psychogenic, or mixed erectile dysfunction.[31]

Adverse events were mild to moderate, the most common being headache, flushing, and nasal congestion (Table 7-5).[29] The monthly rates of headache and dyspepsia, but not flushing, waned with time or were stable (Figure 7-7).[29,30]

Generally, patients with diabetes and erectile dysfunction have a lower response to PDE 5 inhibitors. In a phase III study of 452 erectile dysfunction patients with type 1 or 2 diabetes mellitus,[32] the response rate was high and dose dependent. On general assessment questions, 72% of diabetic men with erectile dysfunction who were taking the 20-mg dose reported improved erections, compared with 57% on 10 mg and 13% on placebo (Figure 7-8). Erectile function, which includes the ability to penetrate and maintain erection, also significantly improved at both doses compared with placebo. Vardenafil, which is now being studied in other patient populations, seems to be a promising alternative to sildenafil.

Tadalafil

Tadalafil (Cialis®), a new, long-acting PDE 5 inhibitor (Figure 7-2), has demonstrated a high selectivity for PDE 5 enzyme in in vitro studies.[33]

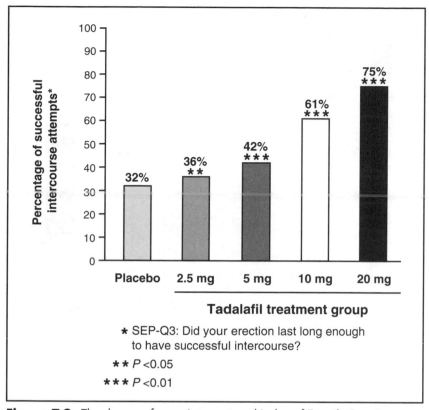

Figure 7-9: The change of mean International Index of Erectile Function erectile function domain scores in a tadalafil clinical trial. Used with permission, Brock et al.[37] SEP-Q3 = Sexual Encounter Profile, question 3.

The most notable differences between sildenafil, vardenafil, and tadalafil are tadalafil's long half-life of 17.5 hours and its lack of visual side effects.[33,34]

A number of clinical studies have been reported on various aspects of tadalafil. To examine the time to onset of response, a three-arm study was conducted in 223 men randomly assigned to placebo, tadalafil 10 mg, or tadalafil 20 mg. The earliest time that tadalafil was significantly superior to placebo was 16 minutes after a 20-mg dose. At 30 minutes, 52% of men tak-

ing 20 mg of tadalafil and 38% of men taking 10 mg of tadalafil developed an erection sufficient for intercourse.[35]

The duration of therapeutic effects of tadalafil was investigated at 24 and 36 hours after dosing in a multicenter, randomized, double-blinded, placebo-controlled, parallel-group study of 348 men (mean age 57 years) with erectile dysfunction.[36] Patients were stratified by baseline severity of erectile dysfunction using the Erectile Function domain score of the International Index of Erectile Function (IIEF) and

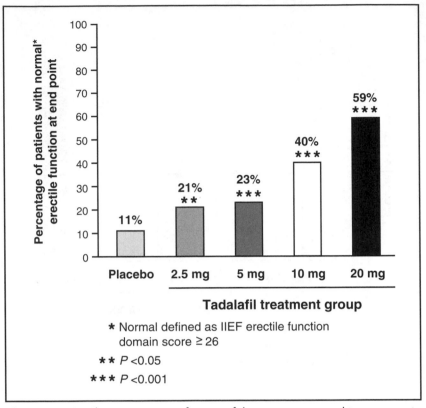

Figure 7-10: The percentage of successful attempts at sexual intercourse in the same tadalafil clinical trial shown in Figure 7-9. Used with permission, Brock et al.[37] IIEF = International Index of Erectile Function.

then randomly allocated within the severity group to receive tadalafil 20 mg (n=175) or placebo (n=173). Subsequently, participants were randomly assigned to two 4-week treatment intervals, during which they were requested to attempt sexual intercourse approximately 24 or 36 hours after tadalafil or placebo dosing. The primary outcome measure was the percentage of successful sexual intercourse attempts (completed to ejaculation), according to patient self-reports using the Sexual Encounter Profile (SEP) diary.

Of the 348 patients, 327 (94%) completed the trial (163 of 175 in the tadalafil group and 164 of 173 in the placebo group). According to the package insert, 36 hours after taking tadalafil, 64% of intercourse attempts were successful vs 37% in the placebo group ($P < 0.001$). The percentage of successful intercourse attempts at about 24 hours after treatment was also significantly greater with tadalafil (61%) than with placebo (37%, $P < 0.001$).

An integrated analysis of five randomized, double-blind, placebo-con-

Table 7-6: Summary of Most Commonly Reported Adverse Events and Discontinuations From Treatment

Safety Variable	Placebo	All Tadalafil	Tadalafil (mg)	
			10	20
No. of patients	308	804	321	258
No. overall safety (%):				
Subjects with >1 treatment emergency adverse event	159 (52)	479 (60)	185 (58)	188 (73)
Discontinuations from adverse events	4 (1.3)	17 (2.1)	5 (1.6)	8 (3.1)
No. most common treatment emergency adverse events (%):				
Headache	19 (6)	114 (4)	37 (12)	55 (21)
Dyspepsia	7 (2)	81 (10)	28 (9)	45 (17)
Back pain	15 (5)	50 (6)	20 (6)	22 (9)
Rhinitis (nasal congestion)	12 (4)	40 (5)	18 (6)	12 (5)
Myalgia	6 (2)	38 (5)	16 (5)	18 (7)
Vasodilatation	6 (2)	30 (4)	11 (3)	14 (5)

No alterations of color vision were reported.

Used with permission, Brock et al.[37]

trolled phase III trials enrolling 1,112 men in 74 centers confirmed the efficacy and safety of tadalafil.[37] The mean age of these men was 59 years (range 22 to 82). Men with mild (41%), moderate (23%), or severe (36%) erectile dysfunction of various etiologies were randomized to placebo or to tadalafil, taken as desired without food or alcohol restrictions, at fixed daily doses of 2.5 mg, 5 mg, 10 mg, or 20 mg. Of these men, 61% had organic dysfunction, 31% had mixed dysfunction, and 8% had psychogenic dysfunction. The three outcome measures were based on changes in the erectile function domain of the IIEF, the SEP, and a global assessment question (GAQ). The two SEP questions were question 2, "Were you able to insert your penis into your partner's vagina?" and question 3, "Did your erection last long enough for you to have successful intercourse?" Compared with placebo, tadalafil (5 to 20 mg) significantly enhanced all efficacy outcomes. Patients receiving 20 mg of tadalafil had a significant im-

Table 7-7: Comparison of the Three PDE Inhibitors

	Sildenafil (Viagra®)	Vardenafil (Levitra®)	Tadalafil (Cialis®)
Efficacy	Excellent	Excellent	Excellent
Onset of action	15 min to 1 h	15 min to 1 h	15 min to 2 h
Half-life	4 h	4-5 h	17.5 h
Therapeutic window	4 to 8 h	4 to 8 h	Up to 36 h
Bioavailability	40%	15%	Not tested
Fatty food	Absorption reduced 29%	Absorption reduced 18%-50%	No effect
Recommended dosage (mg)	25, 50, 100	5, 10, 20	5, 10, 20
Side effects			
Headache, dyspepsia, facial flushing	Yes	Yes	Yes
Backache, myalgia	Rare	Rare	3%-6%
Blurred/blue vision	Yes	Rare	Rare
α-Adrenergic blocker use	Precaution	Contra-indicated	Precaution
Nitrate contraindication	Yes	Yes	Yes

PDE = phosphodiesterase

provement of 7.9 in IIEF erectile function domain score from baseline (P <0.001 vs placebo) and successfully completed 75% of intercourse attempts (SEP question 3) (P <0.001 vs placebo). Improved erections at end point were reported by 81% of the 20-mg tadalafil group and 35% of the control group (P <0.001) (Figures 7-9 and 7-10). The reported side effects included headache, dyspepsia, back pain, rhinitis, myalgia, and flushing (Table 7-6).

Because some oral agents for erectile dysfunction have vasodilatory properties, Kloner et al[38] performed interaction studies between tadalafil and commonly prescribed antihypertensive agents. They also assessed cardiovascular safety using a safety database of phase III studies comparing patients who were and who were not receiving antihypertensives. In patients receiving concomitant antihypertensive therapy, tadalafil administration may result in a reduction in blood pressure that is generally mild and not likely to be of clinical concern. In the phase III studies, no statistically significant differences were observed between tadalafil and placebo in the mean changes in blood pressure from baseline in patients taking two or more antihypertensive agents. The incidence rates of cardiovascular events were comparable between patients who were and those who were not treated with concomitant antihypertensive therapy, with the exception of events recorded as hypertension, which would be expected to occur periodically in this patient population despite treatment. Hypotension or postural hypotension was not reported in any tadalafil-treated patient, compared with one report of each in the placebo-treated patients. Syncope was reported in one tadalafil-treated patient (0.1%) who was not on concomitant antihypertensive medication and in two patients (1.9%) who received placebo with concomitant antihypertensive agents. The results suggest that tadalafil is safe in patients receiving one or more concomitant antihypertensive agents.

In another report examining the effects of tadalafil on the cardiovascular system, safety assessments were performed on a database of >4,000 subjects who received tadalafil in >60 clinical pharmacology, phase II, phase III, and open-label studies.[39] In patients with coronary artery disease (CAD), tadalafil administration before nitrate administration resulted in small decreases in blood pressure. The resulting mean maximal change in standing systolic blood pressure (SBP) after coadministration of sublingual nitroglycerin in patients with chronic stable angina was -36 mm Hg for tadalafil 5 mg, -31 mm Hg for tadalafil 10 mg, and -28 mm Hg for placebo. In addition, a larger number of men had a standing SBP <85 mm Hg after coadministration of sublingual nitroglycerin and tadalafil 5 mg (P <0.001 vs placebo) or tadalafil 10 mg (P <0.01 vs placebo) compared with coadministration with placebo. In patients with chronic stable angina who were taking isosorbide mononitrate on a long-term basis, the mean maximal change in standing SBP was -23 mm Hg for placebo, -23 mm Hg for tadalafil 5 mg, and -26 mm Hg for tadalafil 10 mg. In a study of older subjects ($\geq$55 years) with no overt evidence of CAD, the resulting mean maximal change in standing SBP after coadministration of sublingual nitroglycerin was -25 mm Hg for tadalafil 10 mg, -29 mm Hg for sildenafil 50 mg, and -25 mm Hg for placebo. Cardiac mortality rates in tadalafil studies are consistent with the expected rate in this male population. Across all studies, the incidence rate of myocardial infarction was low in tadalafil-treated patients (0.43 per 100 patient-years) compared with patients who received placebo (0.6 per 100 patient-years), and the incidence rate was comparable to that observed in the age-standardized male population (0.60 per 100 patient-years). The incidence rate of presumed thrombotic strokes in tadalafil studies (0.27 per 100 patient-years) is comparable to the expected rate in this patient population.

The data suggest that tadalafil can be safely used by patients with cardiovascular diseases. As with sildenafil, the use of tadalafil is contraindicated in patients receiving nitrate therapy because of the potential for significant hypotensive effects.

The time course of nitrate interaction was also studied in 150 men after receiving seven consecutive daily doses of placebo or tadalafil (20 mg).[40] On day 7 and beyond, subjects received repeated doses of sublingual nitroglycerin (0.4 mg) after the last dose of placebo or tadalafil. After a 10- to 21-day washout period, subjects crossed over to either placebo or tadalafil, and nitrate dosing was repeated. In response to nitroglycerin at 4, 8, and 24 hours, the following hemodynamic parameters changed significantly with tadalafil: standing systolic blood pressure (SBP) fell below 85 mm Hg, standing diastolic blood pressure (DBP) <45 mm Hg, decrease in SBP >30 mm Hg, and decrease in DBP >20 mm Hg. However, no significant difference was seen at 48, 72, or 96 hours (P >0.49). Nevertheless, as with the other PDE 5 inhibitors, tadalafil should not be administered in combination with organic nitrates.[40]

In clinical trials with tadalafil, two groups of erectile dysfunction patients have had the lowest response rate to this agent: those with diabetes mellitus and those after radical prostatectomy. In one study, men with type 1 or type 2 diabetes and erectile dysfunction were randomly assigned to one of three groups: placebo (n=71), tadalafil 10 mg (n=73), or tadalafil 20 mg (n=72) taken up to once daily for 12 weeks.[41] The co-primary outcome measures were changes from baseline in mean scores on the erectile function domain of the IIEF and changes from baseline in the proportion of "yes" responses to SEP question 2, "Was the patient able to penetrate his partner's vagina?" and SEP question 3, "Was the patient able to complete intercourse?" A total of 191 (88%) of 216 patients completed the study. Treatment with tadalafil significantly improved all primary efficacy variables, regardless of baseline HbA_{1c} level. Therapy with tadalafil also significantly improved a number of secondary outcome measures, including changes in other IIEF domains, individual IIEF questions, and percentage of positive responses to a GAQ measuring erection improvement.

Another study examined the effect of tadalafil in men after bilateral nerve-sparing radical prostatectomy. A total of 303 men (mean age 60 years), 12 to 48 months after surgery, were randomized to receive either tadalafil (n=201) or placebo (n=102). The results of the three co-primary end points were: IIEF, placebo 13, tadalafil 18; SEP question 2, placebo 32%, tadalafil 54%; and SEP question 3, placebo 19%, tadalafil 41%. Tadalafil appeared to be efficacious and well tolerated in these post prostatectomy patients.[42] A comparison of the three PDE 5 inhibitors is shown in Table 7-7.

Comparison of the Three PDE 5 Inhibitors

Although there are major differences among the three PDE 5 inhibitors, no data are available of direct head-to-head study comparing their efficacy. However, several patient preference studies have been published. In a study conducted by Govier et al[43] at 13 sites in the United States and Germany, 215 men with ED were randomized to a double-blind, fixed-dose, 2-period crossover trial with 20 mg of tadalafil and 50 mg of sildenafil. Among these patients, 84.7% were sildenafil naïve and 15.3% had undergone a previous inadequate trial of sildenafil. Of 190 evaluable patients, 126 (66.3%) preferred to initiate treatment with tadalafil, compared with 64 (33.7%) with sildenafil. Interestingly, patients' preferences did not differ by age, duration of ED, treatment sequence, or previous sildenafil exposure. Both medications were well tolerated, with no significant differences in the incidence of treatment-emergent adverse events.

In a report by von Keitz et al,[44] the study design was similar to the Govier et al trial except that the dose of sildenafil was flexible. The study was conducted at 15 sites in Germany, Spain, and the United States, and 219 patients were enrolled. Of the 181 evaluable patients, 132 (73%) chose to receive tadalafil during the extension period. In the dose-titrating assessment, 24 of 36 (67%) preferred tadalafil with tadalafil dosing instructions.

A third study was conducted by Stroberg and associates[45] at 6 sites in Sweden and Italy. The study was a short-term, multicenter, open-label, 1-way crossover trial in patients then taking sildenafil. The goal was to determine how many patients elected to resume sildenafil treatment after a period of treatment with tadalafil vs. continuing with tadalafil therapy. Of the 147 patients who completed the study, 133 (90.5%) elected to take tadalafil in the 6-month extension phase and 14 (9.5%) elected to resume sildenafil. Again, the proportion preferring tadalafil over sildenafil was similar irrespective of age, severity of ED, and sildenafil dose at study entry.

An accompanying commentary with the von Keitz study discussed the study's limitations. Here is a summary of the comments from Ian Eardley and Francesco Montorsi: (1) the comparison of 20 mg of tadalafil to variable dose of sildenafil was inappropriate; (2) the 35% patient limit on patients who were able to titrate to the top dose of sildenafil was unfair; (3) the information sheets demonstrated bias in favor of tadalafil; (4) the use of treatment-naïve patients would have been preferable; (5) food interaction can be avoided in sildenafil or vardenafil if taken 1 hour before eating; and (6) following the proper instructions according to each drug's characteristics is the key to maximizing the success of ED treatment.

In my opinion, having three PDE 5 drugs available for ED patients is most welcome. I have a number of patients who want to try all three drugs before deciding which one suits them the best. These patients want to compare duration of administration, spontaneity, faster onset, a particular side effect, strength of erections, economics, food interaction, lifestyle effects, and drug interactions. While the drug companies are engaged in fierce competition to increase market share, our patients and society benefit from competitive pricing and the availability of three choices. In addition, media attention has clearly increased public awareness of ED as a symptom of many underlying diseases, thus encouraging more patients to seek out consultation with their physicians.

Transdermal and Transurethral Medications

The high drop-out rate from intracavernous injection therapy prompted researchers to seek alternate routes of delivering vasoactive drugs into the corpus cavernosum. For many years, nitroglycerin, a smooth-muscle relaxant, has been used in a paste or cream form for angina. Clinical trials of nitroglycerin paste conducted in the laboratory demonstrated a better erectile response to nitroglycerin than to placebo.[46]

Two alprostadil (PGE$_1$)-based topical agents are now in phase II/III clinical trials. Topiglan™ is alprostadil in combination with SEPA™. Alprox-TD™ is alprostadil in combination with NexACT™. The latter was approved for marketing in China in February 2001 under the name Befar™. These topical agents require milligram dosages (mg) of alprostadil rather than the microgram (μg) dosages used with intracavernous injection. The efficacy and side effects are similar to those of transurethral alprostadil, described below.

Transurethral administration of prostaglandin E$_2$ induced full tumescence in 30% of patients and partial tumescence in 40% of patients.[47] Subsequently, the alprostadil Medicated Urethral System for Erection (MUSE®, PGE$_1$) (Figure 7-11) was also found to be effective. In a large clinical trial, transurethral alprostadil was used in 1,511 patients 26 to 88 years old with chronic erectile dysfunction from various organic causes, with doses ranging from 250 μg to 1,000 μg.[48] During the dose-escalation phase, 66% responded with adequate erection. Of those, 65% had at least one successful intercourse at home, compared with 18% of those taking placebo (Table 7-8). A European study of 249 men showed an overall efficacy of 44%. Side effects reported by more than 2% of patients are listed in Table 7-9. In addition, fibrosis (including curvature, nodules, and Peyronie's plaque) was observed in 1.4% of subjects, and priapism was reported in less than 1%.

This treatment was approved by the FDA in 1996. Because transurethral application is an indirect approach, the patient is advised to sit down or stand up for 10 minutes after application to increase penile venous resistance and thus decrease systemic absorption. To improve clinical efficacy, an adjustable constriction device (Actis®) also may be used. This is placed at the base of the penis to facilitate drug absorption and transport from the corpus spongiosum to the cavernosum.

Prostaglandin E$_1$ is normally present in semen. In 10 normal volunteers, endogenous PGE$_1$ levels in the ejaculate averaged 31 μg (range 0 to 161 μg). In these 10 men, an average of 123 μg of additional PGE$_1$ (range 30 to 369 μg) was present in the ejaculate obtained 10 minutes after administration of 1,000 μg of MUSE®. Because alprostadil has been shown to be embryotoxic when administered subcutaneously to pregnant rats, MUSE® should not be used if the female partner is pregnant, unless a condom is used. Other contraindications are (1) known hypersensitivity to alprostadil; (2) abnormal or inflammatory penile and urethral disease; and (3) sickle cell anemia or trait, thrombocythemia, polycythemia, or multiple myeloma.

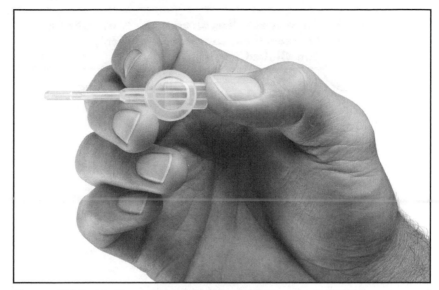

Figure 7-11: Medicated Urethral System for Erection (MUSE®), courtesy of Vivus Inc.

The advantage of transurethral therapy is local administration, minimizing the potential for systemic side effects and drug interaction. The half-life of alprostadil in humans is short, varying between 30 seconds and 10 minutes, depending on the body component in which it is measured and the physiologic status of the subject. Nearly all of the alprostadil entering the central venous circulation is removed in a single pass through the lungs; thus, peripheral venous plasma levels of

Table 7-8: Effect of Transurethral Alprostadil (MUSE®) in Patients With Organic Erectile Dysfunction		
During titration phase (n=1,511)		
	Placebo	*Alprostadil*
Developed adequate erection	NA	65.9%
At-home treatment (n=996)		
	Placebo	*Alprostadil*
Number of patients	500	461
Successful intercourse	18.6%	64.9%

Table 7-9: Adverse Events Reported by >2% of Patients on Transurethral Alprostadil (MUSE®) During Clinical Trials

Adverse Event	% of Patients Reporting	
	MUSE® (n=486)	Placebo (n=511)
Patients		
Penile pain	32	3
Urethral burning	12	4
Urethral bleeding/spotting	5	1
Testicular pain	5	1
Flu symptoms	4	2
Headache	3	2
Infection	3	2
Pelvic pain	2	<1
Dizziness	2	<1
Partners		
Vaginal burning/itching	5.8	0.8

PGE_1 are low or undetectable after MUSE® administration.

The advances in erectile physiology research have helped identify many pharmacologic treatments capable of initiating and enhancing penile erection in patients with erectile dysfunction. However, the simplicity and increased efficacy of these therapies also yield the possibilities of abuse and recreational use. Therefore, most erectile dysfunction experts recommend that these approved first-line therapies (topical, transurethral, and oral agents) should be given only after the physician has obtained a detailed medical and psychosexual history, performed a thorough physical examination and appropriate laboratory tests, established diagnosis, and discussed various diagnostic and treatment options with the patient (and partner, if available).

References

1.   Traish AM, Netsuwan N, Daley J, et al: A heterogeneous population of alpha 1 adrenergic receptors mediates contraction of human corpus cavernosum smooth muscle to norepinephrine. *J Urol* 1995; 153:222-227.

2.   Traish AM, Moreland RB, Huang YH, et al: Expression of functional alpha 2-adrenergic receptor subtypes in human corpus cavernosum and in cultured trabecular smooth muscle cells. *Recept Signal Transduct* 1997;7:55-67.

3.   Hedlund H, Andersson KE: Comparison of the responses to drugs acting on adrenoreceptors and muscarinic recep-

tors in human isolated corpus cavernosum and cavernous artery. *J Auton Pharmacol* 1985;5:81-88.

4. Saenz de Tejada I, Kim N, Lagan I, et al: Regulation of adrenergic activity in penile corpus cavernosum. *J Urol* 1989; 142:1117-1121.

5. Kaplan SA, Reis RB, Kohn IJ, et al: Combination therapy using oral alphablockers and intracavernosal injection in men with erectile dysfunction. *Urology* 1998;52:739-743.

6. Gwinup G: Oral phentolamine in nonspecific erectile insufficiency. *Ann Intern Med* 1988;109:162-163.

7. Goldstein I, and the Vasomax Study Group: Efficacy and safety of oral phentolamine (Vasomax) for the treatment of minimal erectile dysfunction. *J Urol* 1998;159:240.

8. Morales A, Surridge DH, Marshall PG, et al: Nonhormonal pharmacological treatment of organic impotence. *J Urol* 1982;128:45-47.

9. Reid K, Surridge DH, Morales A, et al: Double-blind trial of yohimbine in treatment of psychogenic impotence. *Lancet* 1987;2:421-423.

10. Lal S, Isaac I, Pilapil C, et al: Effect of apomorphine on melatonin secretion in normal subjects. *Prog Neuropsychopharmacol Biol Psychiatry* 1987;11:229-233.

11. Dula E, Bukofzer S, Perdok R, et al: Double-blind, crossover comparison of 3 mg apomorphine SL with placebo and with 4 mg apomorphine SL in male erectile dysfunction. *Eur Urol* 2001;39:558-564.

12. Heaton JP, Morales A, Adams MA, et al: Recovery of erectile function by the oral administration of apomorphine. *Urology* 1995;45:200-206.

13. Saenz de Tejada I, Ware JC, Blanco R, et al: Pathophysiology of prolonged penile erection associated with trazodone use. *J Urol* 1991;145:60-64.

14. Montorsi F, Strambi LF, Guazzoni G, et al: Effect of yohimbine-trazodone on psychogenic impotence: a randomized, double-blind, placebo-controlled study. *Urology* 1994;44:732-736.

15. Korenman SG, Viosca SP: Treatment of vasculogenic sexual dysfunction with pentoxifylline. *J Am Geriatr Soc* 1993; 41:363-366.

16. Goldstein I, Lue TF, Padma-Nathan H, et al: Oral sildenafil in the treatment of erectile dysfunction. Sildenafil Study Group. *N Engl J Med* 1998;338:1397-1404.

17. Boolell M, Allen MJ, Ballard SA, et al: Sildenafil: an orally active type 5 cyclic GMP-specific phosphodiesterase inhibitor for the treatment of penile erectile dysfunction. *Int J Impot Res* 1996;8: 47-52.

18. Zippe CD, Jhaveri FM, Klein EA, et al: Role of Viagra after radical prostatectomy. *Urol* 2000;55:241-245.

19. Morales A, Gingell C, Collins M, et al: Clinical safety of oral sildenafil citrate (Viagra) in the treatment of erectile dysfunction. *Int J Impot Res* 1998;10:69-74.

20. Cheitlin MD, Hutter AM Jr, Brindis RG, et al: Use of sildenafil (Viagra) in patients with cardiovascular disease. Technology and Practice Executive Committee. *Circulation* 1999;99:168-177.

21. Bischoff E, Niewoehner U, Haning H, et al: Vardenafil, a new PDE 5 inhibitor, increases cGMP in rabbit corpus cavernosum. *Int J Impot Res* 2000;12 (suppl 3):A24.

22. Bischoff E, Niewoehner U, Haning H, et al: Vardenafil a potent and selective inhibitor of phosphodiesterase type 5 increases cGMP in rabbit corpus cavernosum. *Int J Impot Res* 2000;13:P40.

23. Saenz de Tejada I, Bischoff E, Niewohner U, et al: Potentiation of the NO-mediated relaxation of human trabecular penile smooth muscle by the PDE 5 inhibitor, vardenafil. Poster presentation at the European Association of Urology, 2001.

24. Saenz de Tejada I, Angulo J, Cuevas P, et al: The phosphodiesterase inhibitory selectivity and the in vitro and in vivo potency of the new PDE5 inhibitor vardenafil. *Int J Impot Res* 2001;13:282-290.

25. Klotz T, Sachse R, Heidrich A, et al: Vardenafil increases penile rigidity and tumescence in erectile dysfunction patients: a RigiScan and pharmacokinetic study. *World J Urol* 2001;19:32-39.

26. Stark S, Sachse R, Liedl T, et al: Vardenafil increases penile rigidity and tumescence in men with erectile dysfunction after a single oral dose. *Eur Urol* 2001;40:181-190.

27. Steidle C, Feldman R, Lettieru J, et al: Pharmacokinetics of vardenafil (a new PDE 5 inhibitor) in the elderly and subgroup data on efficacy and safety in the elderly patients with erectile dysfunction. Poster presentation at the American Geriatrics Society. Chicago, 2001.

28. Sachse R, Rohde G: Safety, tolerability and pharmacokinetics of multiple dose treatment with the new PDE 5 inhibitor Bay 38-9456. Poster presentation at the European Association of Urology, 2000.

29. Porst H, Rosen R, Padma-Nathan H, et al: The efficacy and tolerability of vardenafil, a new, oral, selective phosphodiesterase type 5 inhibitor, in patients with erectile dysfunction: the first at-home clinical trial. *Int J Impot Res* 2001;13:192-199.

30. Young J, Auerbach S, Porst H, et al: Vardenafil, a new selective PDE 5 inhibitor, significantly improved all IIEF domains in patients with erectile dysfunction and showed a favorable safety profile: results at 4 and 12 weeks. Poster presentation at the American Urological Association, 2001.

31. Porst H, Rosen R, Padma-Nathan H, et al: Vardenafil, a new highly selective PDE 5 inhibitor, improves erectile function irrespective of the baseline severity and etiology of ED or age of patient. European Association of Urology, 2001.

32. Goldstein I, Young J, Fischer J, et al: Vardenafil, a new highly selective PDE5 inhibitor, improves erectile function in patients with diabetes mellitus. Poster presentation at the American Diabetes Association, 2001.

33. Corbin JD, Francis SH: Pharmacology of phosphodiesterase-5 inhibitors. *Int J Clin Pract* 2002;56:453-459.

34. Padma-Nathan H, McMurray JG, Pullman WE, et al, for the IC351 On-Demand Dosing Study Group: On-demand IC351 (Cialis™) enhances erectile function in patients with erectile dysfunction. *Int J Impot Res* 2001;13:2-9.

35. Padma-Nathan H, Rosen RC, Shabsigh R, et al: Cialis (IC351) provides prompt response and extended period of responsiveness for the treatment of men with erectile dysfunction (ED). *J Urol* 2001;165(suppl):224, abstract 923.

36. Porst H, Padma-Nathan H, Giuliano F, et al: Efficacy of tadalafil for the treatment of erectile dysfunction at 24 and 36 hours after dosing: a randomized, controlled trial. *Urology* 2003;62:121-125.

37. Brock GB, McMahon CG, Chen KK, et al: Efficacy and safety of tadalafil for the treatment of erectile dysfunction: results of integrated analyses. *J Urol* 2002;168:1332-1336.

38. Kloner RA, Mitchell M, Emmick JT: Cardiovascular effects of tadalafil in patients on common antihypertensive therapies. *Am J Cardiol* 2003;92(suppl):47M-57M.

39. Kloner RA, Mitchell M, Emmick JT: Cardiovascular effects of tadalafil. *J Am Coll Cardiol* 2003;92(suppl):37M-46M.

40. Kloner RA, Hutter AM, Emmick JT, et al: Time course of the interaction between tadalafil and nitrates. *J Am Coll Cardiol* 2003;42:1855-1860.

41. Saenz de Tejada I, Anglin G, Knight JR, et al: Effects of tadalafil on erectile dysfunction in men with diabetes. *Diabetes Care* 2002;25:2159-2164.

42. Montorsi F, McCullough A, Brock G, et al: Tadalafil in the treatment of erectile dysfunction following bilateral nerve-sparing radical retropubic prostatectomy. *Int J Impot Res* 2003;15:S170. Abstract 21.

43. Govier F, Potempa AJ, Kaufman J, et al: A multicenter, randomized, double-blind, crossover study of patient preference for tadalafil 20 mg or sildenafil citrate 50

mg during initiation of treatment for erectile dysfunction. *Clin Ther* 2003;25(11):2709-2723.

44. von Keitz A, Rajfer J, Segal S, et al: A multicenter, randomized, double-blind, crossover study to evaluate patient preference between tadalafil and sildenafil. *Eur Urol* 2004;45:499-507, discussion 507-509.

45. Stroberg P, Murphy A, Costigan T: Switching patients with erectile dysfunction from sildenafil citrate to tadalafil: results of a European multicenter, open-label study of patient preference. *Clin Ther* 2003;25:2724-2737.

46. Heaton JP, Morales A, Owen J, et al: Topical glyceryltrinitrate causes measurable penile arterial dilation in impotent men. *J Urol* 1990;143:729-731.

47. Wolfson B, Pickett S, Scott NE, et al: Intraurethral prostaglandin E$_2$ cream: a possible alternative treatment for erectile dysfunction. *Urology* 1993;42:73-75.

48. Padma-Nathan H, Hellstrom WJ, Kaiser FE, et al: Treatment of men with erectile dysfunction with transurethral alprostadil. Medicated Urethral System for Erection (MUSE) Study Group. *N Engl J Med* 1997;336:1-7.

Chapter 8

Pharmacotherapy: Intracavernous Injection

D e la Torre was the first to use intracavernous injection with isoxsuprine and obtained a US patent for the procedure in 1978. In 1982, Virag reported the incidental finding of erection induced by intracavernous injection of papaverine.[1] The following year, at the annual meeting of the American Urological Association, Brindley personally demonstrated erection after injection of phenoxybenzamine. Subsequently, Zorgniotti and Lefleur reported their experience in instructing patients in the technique of autoinjection of a mixture of papaverine and phentolamine for home use.[2] In the last decade, intracavernous injection therapy has gradually gained worldwide acceptance. Table 8-1 lists drugs that have been used clinically. Several of the most common are addressed in more detail.

Papaverine

Papaverine is an alkaloid isolated from the opium poppy. Its molecular mechanism of action is its inhibitory effect on phosphodiesterase, leading to increased cyclic adenosine monophosphate (cAMP) and cyclic guanine monophosphate (cGMP) in penile erectile tissue. Papaverine also blocks voltage-dependent calcium channels, thus impairing calcium influx, and may also impair calcium-activated potassium and chloride currents. All these actions relax cavernous smooth muscle and penile vessels. Papaverine is metabolized in the liver, and the plasma half-life is 1 to 2 hours.

Home self-injection has since become popular, with the average dose ranging from 15 mg to 60 mg. Papaverine is very effective in psychogenic and neurogenic impotence but is less effective in vasculogenic impotence. The advantages of papaverine are its low cost and stability at room temperature. The major disadvantages are the higher incidences of priapism (0% to 35%) and corporeal fibrosis (1% to 33%) and occasional elevation of liver enzymes. The high incidence of priapism may partly be attributable to the investigators' learning curve in judging the right dose. The fibrotic change seems to be dose dependent and cumulative, although significant fibrosis after only several injections has been reported.[3] The natural course of the fibrosis is not known: some cases resolved several months after injection was discontinued, but others persisted. Systemic side effects include dizziness, pallor, and cold sweats, which may re-

Table 8-1: Common Intracavernous Agents

Drug	Dose Range	Advantages	Disadvantages/ Side Effects
Papaverine	7.5-60 mg	Low cost	Fibrosis, priapism
		Stable at room temperature	Elevation of liver enzymes
Papaverine + phentolamine	0.1-1 mL	More potent than papaverine alone	Fibrosis, priapism Requires refrigeration
Alprostadil	1-60 µg	Metabolized in penis Priapism rare	Painful erection Relatively expensive
Moxisylyte	10-30 mg	Priapism rare	Less potent
Papaverine + phentolamine + alprostadil	0.1-1 mL	Most potent	Requires refrigeration Fibrosis, priapism

sult from vasovagal reflex or hypotension from its vasodilatory effect in patients with veno-occlusive dysfunction.

α-Adrenergic Antagonists

Phentolamine methylate (Regitine®) is a competitive α-adrenoceptor antagonist with equal affinity for α_1 and α_2 receptors. Systemic hypotension, reflex tachycardia, nasal congestion, and gastrointestinal upset are the most common systemic side effects. Phentolamine has a short plasma half-life (30 minutes). When injected intracorporeally alone, it increases corporeal blood flow but does not result in a significant rise in intracorporeal pressure.

Moxisylyte (thymoxamine) is a competitive blocker of α_1-adrenoceptors. It has a short duration of action and some antihistaminic properties. It is less potent than phentolamine in vitro in relaxing cavernous smooth muscle precontracted by norepinephrine. Clinically, it is less effective than papaverine as a single intracorporeal agent.[4] Because of its shorter duration of action, fewer systemic side effects, and low incidence of priapism, moxisylyte is generally considered a safe intracorporeal agent. The rates of prolonged erection and corporeal fibrosis are significantly less than with papaverine.

Alprostadil (Prostaglandin E_1)

The discovery of prostaglandins traces back to the original observation by Kurzrok and Lieb, who noticed that strips of human uterine muscle contract or relax when exposed to human semen.[5] The substance was later identified as a lipid-soluble acid and was named prostaglandin. Alprostadil refers to the exogenous form of prostaglandin E_1. It causes smooth-muscle relaxation, vasodilation, and inhibition of platelet aggregation. It was used clinically for management of patent ductus arteriosus and peripheral vascular disease before being used for intracavernous injection. Alprostadil is metabolized by the enzyme prostaglandin 15-hydroxydehydrogenase, which exists in human corpus cavernosum.[6] After intracavernous injection, 96% of alprostadil is locally metabolized within 1 hour, and no change in peripheral blood levels has been observed.[7]

Several formulations of alprostadil have been used for intracavernous injection. The pediatric formulation (Prostin® VR) was used first,[8] followed by Caverject®, a lyophilized powder specifically developed for intracavernous injection. With Caverject®, every 20 µg of alprostadil also contains excipients of lactose (172 mg), sodium citrate (47 µg), and benzyl alcohol (8.4 mg). Another is alprostadil alfadex (Edex™), which contains alprostadil in the form of an inclusion compound with alpha-cyclodextrin. Caverject® and Edex™ are available in a self-injection system with prefilled diluent syringe, alprostadil, needles, and alcohol swabs in a patient-friendly plastic case. Caverject® is available in 10-µg and 20-µg vials, while Edex™ is available in 5-, 10-, 20-, and 40-µg vials.

Several studies comparing the effects of alprostadil and papaverine have been reported. Alprostadil had a higher response rate and lower incidence of priapism and fibrosis, but the incidence of painful erection was much higher.

In a review of the published literature, Linet and Neff found that, in doses of 10 µg to 20 µg, alprostadil produced full erections in 70% to 80% of patients with erectile dysfunction.[9] The most frequent side effects are listed in Table 8-2. Systemic side effects rarely occurred.

Vasoactive Intestinal Polypeptide

Vasoactive intestinal polypeptide (VIP), originally isolated from the small intestine, is a potent smooth-muscle relaxant. Researchers believe it is one of the nonadrenergic, noncholinergic (NANC) mediators of erection. VIP causes smooth-muscle relaxation and accumulation of cAMP. Intracorporeal injection of VIP does not produce a rigid erection.[10]

Calcitonin Gene-Related Peptide

Calcitonin gene-related peptide (CGRP) is a potent vasodilator. Immunohistochemical techniques have localized CGRP in cavernous nerves, within the walls of cavernous arteries, and in cavernous smooth muscle.[11] CGRP injection induces a dose-related increase in penile inflow. Systemic side effects include facial flushing and hypotension.

Nitric Oxide Donors
Linsidomine

Linsidomine is an antianginal drug that releases nitric oxide (NO) to stimulate the production of cGMP and thus relax smooth muscle. When injected into the corpus cavernosum, it can produce penile erection with

Table 8-2: Most Frequent Side Effects Reported by 1,861 Patients Treated With Caverject® for up to 18 Months

Event	% of patients
Penile pain	37
Prolonged erection	4
Penile fibrosis	3
Injection site hematoma	3
Injection site ecchymosis	2
Headache	2
Dizziness	1

minimal side effects. Porst compared the effect of 1 mg linsidomine with 20 µg alprostadil in 40 patients with erectile dysfunction and reported that the erectile and hemodynamic response to linsidomine was less than with alprostadil.[12]

Sodium Nitroprusside

Sodium nitroprusside, an NO donor, is an inorganic hypotensive agent. Its main pharmacologic action is the relaxation of vascular smooth muscle. Brock et al reported that intracavernous injection of nitroprusside caused severe hypotension in their first three patients, which prompted discontinuation of a clinical trial.[13] However, Martinez-Pineiro et al performed a study comparing the effect of intracavernous administration of sodium nitroprusside (100 to 400 µg) with alprostadil (20 µg) in 105 patients. They found that nitroprusside induced penile erection in many patients, with insignificant side effects.[14] Nevertheless, they concluded that alprostadil was still a better choice.

Drug Combinations
Papaverine and Phentolamine

Zorgniotti and Lefleur first reported the use of a combination of papaverine (30 mg) and phentolamine (0.5 mg) for self-injection. This was effective in 72% of 250 patients.[2] Prolonged erection occurred in 1.6% of patients during titration and in one patient on home therapy. Fibrosis developed in 4.1% of patients. Stief and Wetterauer compared papaverine or phentolamine alone with a papaverine/phentolamine combination in men with organic erectile dysfunction. They found that full erection occurred in 40% of patients with papaverine alone, in 7% of patients with phentolamine alone, and in 87% of patients with papaverine/phentolamine.[15]

In a study of 160 men with erectile failure by Armstrong et al,[16] 13,030 intracavernous papaverine and phentolamine injections were reported. An erection sufficient for sexual intercourse was achieved in 115 patients (72%). Response rates varied with type of impotence: vasculogenic

(48%), psychogenic (93%), neurogenic (92%), diabetic (68%), idiopathic (63%), traumatic (60%), alcohol-related (80%), and drug-related (75%). After a mean follow-up period of 14.1 months, 55 (48%) were still successfully using intracavernous therapy. A total of 22 episodes of priapism occurred in 16 patients, and 1 patient developed corporeal fibrosis.

Papaverine, Phentolamine, and Alprostadil

Virag et al first used a combination of six drugs (ceritine, which contains atropine, dipyridamole, ifenprodil, papaverine, piribedil, and yohimbine) in treating erectile dysfunction.[17] In 1991, Bennett et al introduced a three-drug mixture containing 2.5 mL papaverine (30 mg/mL), 0.5 mL phentolamine (5 mg/mL), and 0.05 mL alprostadil (500 µg/mL) for intracavernous injection. Theoretically, because each of the three has a different mechanism of action, the combination should be synergistic and permit a much lower dose of each, avoiding the side effects of high doses. They found that 89% of the patients had adequate erection and progressed to home injection therapy.[18]

In another study, 32 patients who failed alprostadil alone or the dual combination of papaverine/phentolamine had adequate erection with the triple combination.[19] The triple-drug combination is more effective than alprostadil alone and has a much lower incidence of painful erection.

Other Drug Combinations

Floth and Schramek reported that the combination of papaverine (7.5 mg) and alprostadil (5 µg) is more effective than alprostadil alone (10 µg) and might suitably replace papaverine/phentolamine or alprostadil alone in patients who do not respond well or who suffer side effects after high single doses.[20] Montorsi et al used a mixture of 12.1 mg/mL papaverine hydrochloride, 10.1 µg/mL alprostadil, 1.01 mg/mL phentolamine mesylate, and 0.15 mg/mL atropine sulfate in a group of patients with veno-occlusive dysfunction.[21] The mean volume injected was 0.42 ± 0.09 mL (range 0.25 to 0.90 mL). They noted that 95% of patients achieved sustained rigid erections. Gerstenberg et al reported a study of a combination of VIP (30 µg) and phentolamine (0.5 to 2.0 mg) in 52 men with erectile dysfunction.[22] A total of 1,380 self-injections were given. After sexual stimulation, all patients obtained adequate erection. None developed priapism, fibrosis, or systemic side effects. Kiely et al reported that a combination of papaverine and VIP produced penile rigidity similar to that with papaverine and phentolamine.[10] Truss et al reported the result of pharmacologic testing with a mixture of CGRP (5 µg) and alprostadil (10 µg) in 68 patients. Twenty-eight had erectile dysfunction and venous leak and had failed penile venous surgery, another 28 had erectile dysfunction and venous leak but had refused penile venous surgery, and 12 patients had no venous leak but had a poor response to maximal doses of papaverine and phentolamine. Erections sufficient for intercourse occurred in 19 of the 28 patients in the first group (67.9%), 20 patients (71.4%) in the second, and 11 patients (91.7%) in the third.[23]

Other Aspects of Intracavernous Injection Therapy
Efficacy in Different Types of Erectile Dysfunction

In patients with nonvascular causes (eg, psychogenic, hormonal, neurogenic), the response rate to intracavernous injection is very high (80% to 100%). In vascular cases, the rate is considerably lower, and a higher dosage is required. When response is low after repeated testing and sexual stimulation, the most likely diagnosis is severe vascular disease (arterial, venous, or both), although in rare cases psychological inhibition may be strong enough to impair the erectile response.

Improvement in Spontaneous Erection

Many patients experience improvement or recovery of spontaneous erections when practicing self-injection over the long term. Although reduction in performance anxiety may occur in patients with a considerable psychogenic component, several blood flow studies have shown an improvement after long-term intracavernous injection.[24]

Patient Acceptance and Drop-Out Rate

In several studies, the percentage of patients accepting injection therapy when offered in the office ranges from 49% to 84%.[25,26] The reasons for declining therapy include penile pain, inadequate response, fear of the needle, unnaturalness, and loss of sex drive. In long-term studies, 13% to 60% of patients drop out. Their reasons include loss of interest, loss of partner, poor erectile response, penile pain, concomitant illness, recovery of spontaneous erection, and ultimate choice of other therapy.

Serious Adverse Effects

Priapism and fibrosis are the two more serious side effects associated with intracavernous injection therapy. Linet and Neff calculated that priapism occurred in 1.3% of 8,090 patients in 48 studies with alprostadil.[9] The incidence was about five times lower with alprostadil than with papaverine or the combination of papaverine and phentolamine (1.5% vs 10% vs 7%). Fibrosis can occur as a nodule, diffuse scarring, a plaque, or curvature. The incidence is about 10 times lower with alprostadil than with papaverine or papaverine/phentolamine (1% vs 12% vs 9% of patients), although one study reported a 12% incidence with alprostadil.

Dosage and Administration

The first injection must be performed by medical personnel, and patients must receive appropriate training and education before home injection. For alprostadil, an initial dose of 2.5 µg is recommended. If the response is inadequate, increases in 2.5-µg increments can be given until a full erection is achieved or a maximum of 60 µg is reached.

As a general rule, patients should start with a small dose (eg, 7.5 mg of papaverine, 0.1 mL of combination drugs), especially in patients with nonvascular erectile dysfunction. The goal is to achieve an erection that is adequate for sexual intercourse but lasts for less than 1 hour. Patients who use excessive amounts to maintain erection for more than 1 hour may require increasing doses to achieve and maintain the same erection and eventually may fail to achieve erection at all.

Contraindications

Intracavernous injection therapy is contraindicated in patients with sickle cell anemia, schizophrenia or other severe psychiatric disorders, severe venous incompetence, or severe systemic disease. In patients taking an anticoagulant or aspirin, compressing the injection site for 7 to 10 minutes after injection is recommended. In patients with poor manual dexterity or poor eyesight, the sexual partner can be instructed to perform the injection. The clinician may wish to consult a medical ethics committee if the patient has an active venereal disease or other infectious disease, a history of sexual violence, or a conviction for a sex offense.

Future of Intracavernous Injection: Gene Therapy?

The advance in molecular biology and the better understanding of neurophysiology of penile erection have opened a new front in the battle against erectile dysfunction. The elucidation of NO-cGMP-ion channels as the physiologic pathway leading to penile erection has enabled researchers to manipulate this pathway for possible cure of erectile dysfunction. The external location of the penis, the large smooth muscle content, and the feasibility of applying a tourniquet at the base for up to half an hour make the penis one of the ideal organs for gene and growth factor therapy by intracavernous injection. Garban et al[27] first reported transfecting iNOS gene and subsequently nNOS gene to the penile tissue to enhance penile erection in old rats. Champion et al[28] transfected penile tissue of aged rats with eNOS gene carried by adenovirus and also showed improved erections. Christ and Melman[29] injected plasmid containing naked DNA of potassium channels to the penis of diabetic rats and demonstrated a significant improvement in erection. In a different approach, Wessells and Williams[30] transplanted fluorescently labeled autologous microvessel endothelial cells into the rat corpus cavernosum. They were able to show that transplanted endothelial cells adhere and persist in the corporal sinusoids and provide a rationale for cell-based gene therapy in the penis. In our laboratory, we have tried a different approach aiming at restoring the degenerated nerves, arteries, and cavernous smooth muscles by injecting into the rat penis growth factor protein or growth factor genes carried by adeno-associated virus. We have complete successes in restoring erections in moderate arteriogenic, hyperlipidemic, and castration-induced erectile dysfunction models.[31,32] Partial successes were obtained in severe arteriogenic and irradiation-induced erectile dysfunction models. Because of the potential for a 'cure' with the aforementioned therapies, intracavernous injection may become the preferred treatment for erectile dysfunction in the future.

References

1. Virag R: Intracavernous injection of papaverine for erectile failure. *Lancet* 1982;2:938.

2. Zorgniotti AW, Lefleur RS: Auto-injection of the corpus cavernosum with a vasoactive drug combination for vasculogenic impotence. *J Urol* 1985;133:39-41.

3. Corriere JN Jr, Fishman IJ, Benson GS, et al: Development of fibrotic penile

lesions secondary to the intracorporeal injection of vasoactive agents. *J Urol* 1988; 140:615-617.

4. Buvat J, Lemaire A, Marcolin G, et al: Intracavernous injections of vasoactive drugs. Evaluation of their diagnostic and therapeutic value in 65 cases of erectile impotence. *J Urol (Paris)* 1986;92:111-116.

5. Kurzrok R, Lieb CC: Biochemical studies of human semen. II. The action of semen on the human uterus. *Proc Soc Exp Biol Med* 1930;28:268.

6. Roy AC, Adaikan PG, Sen DK, et al: Prostaglandin 15-hydroxydehydrogenase activity in human penile corpora cavernosa and its significance in prostaglandin-mediated penile erection. *Br J Urol* 1989; 64:180-182.

7. van Ahlen H, Peskar BA, Sticht G, et al: Pharmacokinetics of vasoactive substances administered into the human corpus cavernosum. *J Urol* 1994;151:1227-1230.

8. Stackl W, Hasun R, Marberger M: Intracavernous injection of prostaglandin E_1 in impotent men. *J Urol* 1988;140: 66-68.

9. Linet OI, Neff LL: Intracavernous prostaglandin E_1 in erectile dysfunction. *Clin Investig* 1994;72:139-149.

10. Kiely EA, Bloom SR, Williams G: Penile response to intracavernosal vasoactive intestinal polypeptide alone and in combination with other vasoactive agents. *Br J Urol* 1989;64:191-194.

11. Stief CG, Benard F, Bosch RJ, et al: A possible role for calcitonin-gene-related peptide in the regulation of the smooth muscle tone of the bladder and penis. *J Urol* 1990;143:392-397.

12. Porst H: Prostaglandin E_1 and the nitric oxide donor linsidomine for erectile failure: a diagnostic comparative study of 40 patients. *J Urol* 1993;149:1280-1283.

13. Brock G, Breza J, Lue TF, et al: Intracavernous sodium nitroprusside: inappropriate impotence treatment. *J Urol* 1993;150:864-867.

14. Martinez-Pineiro L, Lopez-Tello J, Alonso Dorrego JM, et al: Preliminary results of a comparative study with intracavernous sodium nitroprusside and prostaglandin E_1 in patients with erectile dysfunction. *J Urol* 1995;153:1487-1490.

15. Stief CG, Wetterauer U: Erectile responses to intracavernous papaverine and phentolamine: comparison of single and combined delivery. *J Urol* 1988; 140:1415-1416.

16. Armstrong DK, Convery A, Dinsmore WW: Intracavernosal papaverine and phentolamine for the medical management of erectile dysfunction in a genitourinary clinic. *Int J STD AIDS* 1993;4:214-216.

17. Virag R, Shoukry K, Floresco J, et al: Intracavernous self-injection of vasoactive drugs in the treatment of impotence: 8-year experience with 615 cases. *J Urol* 1991;145:287-293.

18. Bennett AH, Carpenter AJ, Barada JH: An improved vasoactive drug combination for a pharmacological erection program. *J Urol* 1991;146:1564-1565.

19. Goldstein I, Borges FD, Fitch WP, et al: Rescuing the failed papaverine/phentolamine erection: a proposed synergistic action of papaverine, phentolamine, and PGE_1. *J Urol* 1990;143:304A.

20. Floth A, Schramek P: Intracavernous injection of prostaglandin E_1 in combination with papaverine: enhanced effectiveness in comparison with papaverine plus phentolamine and prostaglandin E_1 alone. *J Urol* 1991;145:56-59.

21. Montorsi F, Guazzoni G, Bergamaschi F, et al: Four-drug intracavernous therapy for impotence due to corporeal veno-occlusive dysfunction. *J Urol* 1993;149:1291-1295.

22. Gerstenberg TC, Metz P, Ottesen B, et al: Intracavernous self-injection with vasoactive intestinal polypeptide and phentolamine in the management of erectile failure. *J Urol* 1992;147:1277-1279.

23. Truss MC, Becker AJ, Thon WF, et al: Intracavernous calcitonin gene-related peptide plus prostaglandin E_1: possible alternative to penile implants in selected patients. *Eur Urol* 1994;26:40-45.

24. Marshall GA, Breza J, Lue TF: Improved hemodynamic response after long-term intracavernous injection for impotence. *Urology* 1994;43:844-848.

25. Chandeck Montesa K, Chen Jimenez J, Tamayo JC, et al: Prospective study of the effectiveness and side effects of intracavernous prostaglandin E_1 versus papaverine or papaverine phentolamine in the diagnosis and treatment of erection dysfunction. Review of the literature. *Actas Urol Esp* 1992;16:208-216.

26. Gerber GS, Levine LA: Pharmacological erection program using prostaglandin E_1. *J Urol* 1991;146:786-789.

27. Garban H, Marquez D, Magee T, et al: Cloning of rat and human inducible penile nitric oxide synthase. Application for gene therapy of erectile dysfunction. *Biol Reprod* 1997;56:954-963.

28. Champion HC, Bivalacqua TJ, Hyman AL, et al: Gene transfer of endothelial nitric oxide synthase to the penis augments erectile responses in the aged rat. *Proc Natl Acad Sci U S A* 1999;96: 11648-11652.

29. Christ GJ, Melman A: The application of gene therapy to the treatment of erectile dysfunction. *Int J Impot Res* 1998;10:111-112.

30. Wessells H, Williams SK: Endothelial cell transplantation into the corpus cavernosum: moving towards cell-based gene therapy. *J Urol* 1999;162:2162-2164.

31. Bakircioglu ME, Lin CS, Fan P, et al: The effect of adeno-associated virus mediated brain derived neurotrophic factor in an animal model of neurogenic impotence. *J Urol* 2001;165:2103-2109.

32. Lee MC, El-Sakka AI, Graziottin TM, et al: The effect of vascular endothelial growth factor on a rat model of traumatic arteriogenic erectile dysfunction. *J Urol* 2002;167:761-767.

Chapter 9

External Erection Device

The vacuum constriction device is an effective and safe treatment for erectile dysfunction. It consists of a plastic cylinder connected directly or by tubing to a vacuum-generating source—a manually-operated or battery-operated pump (Figure 9-1). After the penis is engorged by the negative pressure, a constricting ring is applied to the base to maintain the erection. To avoid injury, the ring should not be left in place for more than 30 minutes. In an animal experiment, a negative intracavernous pressure was recorded in the corpus cavernosum immediately after a wall suction was applied to the penis. This was followed by engorgement of all components of the penis, including corpora cavernosa, corpus spongiosum, glans, and venous channels. Release of the suction resulted in rapid detumescence unless a constriction device was placed at the base of the penis to trap blood in the penis.

The erection produced by a vacuum device is different from a physiologic erection or one produced by intracavernous injection. The blood oxygen level in the corpus cavernosum is lower and the portion of the penis proximal to the ring is flaccid, which may produce a pivoting effect. The penile skin may be cold and dusky, and ejaculation may be trapped by the constricting ring. The ring can be uncomfortable or even painful. However, in many patients the device can produce an erection that is close to normal and sufficiently rigid for coitus. The device also engorges the glans and is useful for patients with glanular insufficiency.

In patients with severe proximal venous leak, severe arterial insufficiency, or fibrosis secondary to priapism or an infection from a prosthesis, the device may not produce adequate erection. In these cases, combining intracavernous injection with the vacuum constriction device may enhance the erection.[1] The device can also be used successfully by men with a malfunctioning penile prosthesis.[2,3] I have extended the use of the vacuum device for various conditions to prevent shortening of the penis (Table 9-1).

Most men using the device report satisfaction with penile rigidity, length, and circumference; partner satisfaction is likewise high.[4] Patients also report an improvement in self-esteem and sense of well-being. Complications include penile pain and numbness (occasional, 45%; often, 5%), difficult ejaculation (23%), ec-

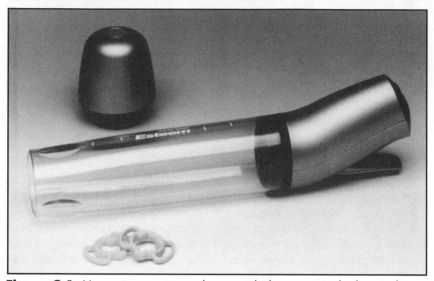

Figure 9-1: Vacuum constriction device with the pump, cylinder, and constriction band. (Courtesy of Timm Medical Technology.)

chymosis and petechiae (32% to 38%), pain or swelling after device use (16% to 28%), and pivoting of penis (35%).[5] Patients taking aspirin or warfarin (Coumadin®) should exercise caution when using these devices (Table 9-2).

Cookson and Nadig reported satisfaction rates from 68% to 83%.[6] In a prospective study of the medical, sexual, and psychosocial outcomes of 29 men regularly using a vacuum device for 6 months, Turner et al reported statistically significant improvements in erectile quality, frequency of intercourse attempts, frequency of orgasm, and sexual satisfaction.[7] The study also showed a decrease in psychiatric symptoms, increased self-esteem, and a trend toward improved marital satisfaction. Many partners reported improved sexual function through increased frequency of orgasm, decreased mas-turbation, and greater sexual satisfaction, with no changes in psychosocial parameters.

The device is more acceptable to older men in a steady relationship than to young single men in search of a partner. It is safe when used properly and is one of the least costly treatment options ($150 to $500). Although it can be used by any patient with erectile dysfunction, we still recommend that a reasonable work-up (including a detailed medical and psychosexual history, physical examination, and appropriate laboratory tests) be conducted so that some easily correctable cause of the dysfunction will not be overlooked.

The devices listed in Table 9-3 have been approved by the Food and Drug Administration for medical use. A safety-release valve is incorporated into the system once the pressure is above 300 to 500 mm Hg to avoid

Table 9-1: Indications for Vacuum Constriction Device

Condition	Rationale
Erectile dysfunction	Helps initiate and maintain erection
Veno-occlusive dysfunction	Helps maintain erection (constriction device may suffice)
After radical prostatectomy	Helps initiate and maintain erection Prevents shortening of penis*
After penile vascular surgery	Prevents shortening of penis*
After removal of prosthesis	Prevents shortening of penis*
After venous grafting for Peyronie's disease	Stretches the graft (tissue expansion)*

*30 min/d stretching by vacuum device without constriction band.

Table 9-2: Relative Contraindications to Vacuum Constriction Device Therapy

Medical	Social
• Sickle cell disease	• Active phase of venereal or infectious disease
• Anticoagulation therapy	• Convicted sex offender
• Bleeding disorder	
• Severe penile deformity	
• Recurrent priapism	

Table 9-3: Vacuum Constriction Devices

Company	Device
Timm Medical Technology	ErecAid, Esteem
Post-T-Vac	Post-T-Vac system
Mentor	Response system
Vetco	VET system
Encore	VTU system

penile injury. Some patients may purchase similar devices from sex shops to save money. Because penile injuries from household vacuum cleaners have been reported, patients should be warned not to use such a high-pressure device.

References

1. Marmar JL, DeBenedictis TJ, Praiss DE: The use of a vacuum constrictor device to augment a partial erection following an intracavernous injection. *J Urol* 1988;140:975-979.

2. Korenman SG, Viosca SP: Use of a vacuum tumescence device in the management of impotence in men with a history of penile implant or severe pelvic disease. *J Am Geriatr Soc* 1992;40:61-64.

3. Sidi AA, Becher EF, Zhang G, et al: Patient acceptance of and satisfaction with an external negative pressure device for impotence. *J Urol* 1990;144:1154-1156.

4. Sidi AA, Lewis JH: Clinical trial of a simplified vacuum erection device for impotence treatment. *Urology* 1992;39: 526-528.

5. Nadig PW: Six years' experience with the vacuum constriction device. *Int J Impot Res* 1989;1:55-58.

6. Cookson MS, Nadig PW: Long-term results with vacuum constriction device. *J Urol* 1993;149:290-294.

7. Turner LA, Althof SE, Levine SB, et al: Treating erectile dysfunction with external vacuum devices: impact upon sexual, psychological and marital functioning. *J Urol* 1990;144:79-82.

Chapter 10

Vascular Surgery

Of the many causes of impotence, vasculogenic dysfunction is believed to be one of the most common. Vasculogenic erectile dysfunction can be categorized into two types: arteriogenic and venogenic (cavernosal). Arteriogenic erectile dysfunction is the inability to produce adequate erection because of insufficient arterial inflow into the penis. Venogenic erectile dysfunction, on the other hand, is the inability to achieve or maintain erection because of a defect in the veno-occlusive mechanism of the penis. This chapter outlines the vascular surgical techniques and principles involved in the treatment of vasculogenic impotence.

Surgery for Arteriogenic Erectile Dysfunction

Patient Selection and Evaluation

Arteriogenic impotence has a variety of etiologies. In many patients with arteriogenic impotence, penile arterial insufficiency is associated with other risk factors that predispose to vascular disease. Risk factors for arteriogenic impotence include diabetes mellitus, hypertension, coronary and generalized vascular disease, and hypercholesterolemia. Because of the multiple risk factors, overlapping causes of impotence, and diffuse nature of the arterial lesions, most older patients with arteriogenic impotence are not candidates for arterial revascularization.

However, a small subset of patients with arteriogenic impotence can benefit from penile arterial revascularization. This group consists mostly of young patients with discrete arterial lesions secondary to traumatic pelvic or perineal injury. In these patients, duplex sonography and cavernosometry and cavernosography should be performed to assess arterial and veno-occlusive function. In addition to locating the site of occlusion, the clinician should also assess the donor vessel (most commonly the inferior epigastric artery) and the recipient vessel (the dorsal artery) by pharmacologic pudendal arteriography.

Surgical Technique

Numerous revascularization techniques are reported in the literature. Our approach is described below. We prefer epigastric to dorsal artery bypass if the angiogram or color duplex ultrasound shows communication between the dorsal and the cavernous arteries. We routinely measure the intraluminal pressure of the epigastric and the dorsal arteries with an arterial line setup. An arterial-arterial bypass is performed only if the pressure in the epigastric artery is 10 mm Hg higher than the dorsal artery. If the pressure difference is less than 10 mm Hg, an epigastric artery-dorsal vein anastomosis is performed.

Dorsal artery revascularization (inferior epigastric artery to dorsal artery of the penis). In 1980, Michal reported the results of penile arterial revascularization using the inferior epigastric artery as the donor vessel anastomosed to the dorsal artery of the penis.[1] This technique relies on collateral circulation from the dorsal artery supplying the corpora cavernosa. Approximately 55% to 80% of patients reported full return of normal erections after this procedure.[1,2] To preserve distal circulation, we prefer harvesting two distal branches from the epigastric artery for the anastomosis to the proximal and distal ends of the dorsal artery. If this is not done, an end-to-side connection is the next procedure of choice.

Dorsal vein arterialization (inferior epigastric artery to deep dorsal vein of the penis). In contrast to revascularization of the dorsal artery, penile arterial flow can also be restored by arterialization of the deep dorsal vein of the penis. Virag reported on his experience with penile arterial revascularization using the inferior epigastric artery as the donor vessel, anastomosed to the deep dorsal vein.[3] The vascular anastomosis is performed at the base of the penis. Virag and Bennett reported that 60% of patients experienced improvement in the quality of their erec-

tion.[4] Several modifications have been reported. Furlow et al reported the results of a modification of the Virag procedure, in which the proximal and distal ends of the deep dorsal vein and contributing tributaries were ligated. We prefer an end-to-side arteriovenous anastomosis at the base of the penis and ligation of the deep dorsal vein proximally and distally. Although some expect that retrograde flow into the sinusoids will provide additional flow, we believe that an increase in venous resistance is the more likely hemodynamic event after the procedure. Dorsal vein arterialization has yielded an overall success rate around 50%.[4-6]

Complications

Complications associated with arterial bypass surgery include hematoma, infection, occlusion of anastomosis, and penile shortening. In epigastric artery-dorsal vein bypass surgery, an incidence of glans hyperemia as high as 10% has been reported. Glans hyperemia can be treated by surgical ligation of the distal end of the dorsal artery or the ligation of veins just proximal to the corona. Other complications include anastomotic thromboses and glans hypoesthesia from injury to the dorsal neurovascular bundle.

Arterial-arterial anastomosis is a more physiologic approach than are arteriovenous procedures and gives better long-term results. Arteriovenous anastomosis usually results in thickening of the dorsal vein and eventual thrombosis of the anastomosis. However, some patients continue to do well, probably because of the decrease in venous return.

Surgery for Venogenic Erectile Dysfunction

Patient Selection and Evaluation

Venogenic erectile dysfunction is the inability to achieve or maintain erection because of the inability to trap blood within the corpora cavernosa. The various causes of veno-occlusive dysfunction have been broadly categorized into the following: (1) ectopic veins; (2) abnormalities of the tunica albuginea (eg, Peyronie's disease); (3) abnormalities of the cavernous smooth muscle, leading to inadequate relaxation (eg, fibrosis secondary to priapism, aging); (4) inadequate neurotransmitter release; and (5) abnormal communication between the corpus cavernosum and spongiosum or glans penis (eg, Winter's shunt[7]).

Venogenic dysfunction is often suspected in the course of impotence evaluation by the finding of a suboptimal erectile response to intracavernous injection despite a normal arterial response on duplex sonography. A persistent end-diastolic flow of greater than 5 cm/sec on duplex sonography also has been shown in some studies to correlate with venous leak. The diagnosis can also be made by dynamic infusion cavernosometry and cavernosography (DICC). Cavernosometry and cavernosography can document the severity of venous leak as well as visualize the site.

Surgical Technique

The complexity of venous drainage of the penis may be key in explaining the lack of long-term success of venous ligation procedures. Multiple venous leak sites can be visualized in most patients. Common leak sites include the superficial and deep dorsal vein, crural veins, corpus spongiosum, and glans penis. Various surgical procedures have been described, aimed at correcting the radiographic finding of venous leak. Although multiple drainage sites and communications may be seen on cavernosography, the deep dorsal vein and the cavernous (crural) veins are the main venous drainage of the corpora cavernosa and are the most common sites for ligation.

Our preferred surgical approach is deep dorsal vein resection and crural ligation.[8] The procedure is performed through an inguinoscrotal incision. After releasing the suspensory ligaments, the penis is detached from the pubic bone. The deep dorsal vein is identified, ligated, and resected. Careful microscopic dissection of the cavernous and dorsal arteries and the dorsal and cavernous nerves is then performed at the hilum of the penis. Once the entrance of the cavernous arteries is identified and the dorsal neurovascular bundle is lifted from the tunica, a urethral catheter is inserted, and a 1-cm segment of the crura isolated. Two umbilical tapes are then looped around each crus and ligated. The penis is then reattached to the periosteum of the pubis with nonabsorbable sutures, and the tissue is closed in layers to prevent penile shortening. If communication between the corpus cavernosum and the spongiosum is identified on cavernosogram, a spongiolysis and individual suture ligation of communications are performed.

Results of Penile Venous Surgery

Despite the promising early results of penile venous surgery, long-term results have been disappointing. Although several researchers have reported short-term success rates of up to 70% in selected patients, longer-term follow-ups show a significant decline.[9,10] Development of venous collateral and persistent venous leak seem to be contributing factors in many patients who fail to improve after venous surgery. Factors that may predict a poor prognosis include increasing patient age, duration of impotence, multiple leak sites, a proximal (crural) venous leak site, and concomitant arteriogenic insufficiency.[11]

Therapeutic options for patients with vasculogenic erectile dysfunction and Peyronie's disease have been greatly broadened by an increased understanding of the pathophysiology of these disorders. Although the role of surgery in the treatment of vasculogenic erectile disorders still remains to be clearly defined, the techniques outlined represent a basis for future innovations.

References

1. Michal V: Revascularization procedures of the cavernous bodies in vasculogenic impotence. In: Zorgniotti A, Rossi G, eds. *Proceedings of the First International Conference of Corpus Cavernosum Revascularization.* Springfield, IL, Charles C. Thomas, 1980, pp 239-255.

2. Goldstein I, Hatzichristou DG, Pescatori EG: Pelvic, perineal, and penile trauma-associated arteriogenic impotence: pathophysiologic mechanisms and the role of microvascular arterial bypass surgery. In: Bennett AH, ed. *Impotence—Diagnosis and Management of Erectile Dysfunction.* Philadelphia, WB Saunders, 1994, pp 213-228.

3. Virag R: Revascularization of the penis. In: Bennett AH, ed. *Management of Male Impotence.* Baltimore, Williams & Wilkins, 1982, pp 219-233.

4. Virag R, Bennett AH: Arterial and venous surgery for vasculogenic impotence: a combined French and American experience. *Arch Ital Urol Nefrol Androl* 1991;63:95-100.

5. Furlow WL, Fisher J, Knoll LD, et al: Current status of penile revascularization with deep dorsal vein arterialization: experience with 95 patients. *Int J Impot Res* 1990;2:348-349.

6. Lizza E, Zorgniotti A: Penile revascularization for impotence: comparison of the V-S and the Furlow operations. *J Urol* 1988;139:298A.

7. Winter CC: Cure of idiopathic priapism: new procedure for creating fistula between glans penis and corpora cavernosa. *Urology* 1976;8:389-391.

8. Lue TF: Treatment of venogenic impotence. In: Tanagho EA, Lue TF, McClure RD, eds. *Contemporary Management of Impotence and Infertility.* Baltimore, Williams & Wilkins, 1988, pp 175-177.

9. Wespes E, Schulman C: Venous impotence: pathophysiology, diagnosis and treatment. *J Urol* 1993;149:1238-1245.

10. Lewis RW: Venogenic impotence: is there a future? *Curr Opin Urol* 1994; 6:340-342.

11. Freedman AL, Costa Neto F, Mehringer CM, et al: Long-term results of penile vein ligation for impotence from venous leakage. *J Urol* 1993;149:1301-1303.

Chapter 11

Penile Prostheses

Before 1983, the insertion of a penile prosthesis was the only effective treatment for organic impotence. Since then, highly effective and minimally invasive therapies such as oral phosphodiesterase type 5 (PDE 5) inhibitor, intracavernous injection, vacuum constriction devices, and transurethral therapy have become the treatment of choice for most patients. Therefore, patients should be informed and should have a chance to try the less invasive alternative therapies before penile prosthesis is offered. Table 11-1 lists indications and contraindications for penile prosthesis.

Types of Penile Prostheses

Penile prostheses are classified into three general types: malleable (semirigid), mechanical, and inflatable devices (Figures 11-1, 11-2, and 11-3; Table 11-2). The malleable devices are made of silicone rubber, and several models contain a central intertwined metallic core. The mechanical device also is made of silicone rubber, but it contains polytetrafluoroethylene-coated interlocking polysulfone rings in a rod column that provides rigidity when the rings are lined up and flaccidity when the penis is bent.[1] Inflatable (hydraulic) devices are further divided into two-piece and

three-piece devices. Two-piece inflatable prostheses consist of a pair of cylinders attached to a scrotal pump-reservoir. There is one two-piece inflatable prosthesis on the market: the AMS Ambicor®. Three-piece inflatable penile prostheses consist of paired penile cylinders, a scrotal pump, and a suprapubic fluid reservoir. Mentor Corp. makes one three-piece inflatable prosthesis (Titan™; regular and narrow-base); American Medical Systems makes four three-piece devices: the AMS 700 CX™, the AMS 700 CXM™, the AMS 700 Ultrex™, and the AMS 700 Ultrex™ Plus. The Ultrex prostheses contain distal expansion mechanisms that can increase length of erection.[2] In the past 2 years, three innovations have been applied to the prosthetic devices: (1) AMS antibiotic coated prosthesis (InhibiZone™), (2) AMS Parylene™ coating to strengthen the cylinder, and (3) Mentor lock-out valve reservoir to prevent autoinflation.

Selection of Penile Prosthesis

Although all the devices yield excellent results for penile rigidity, some patients may do better with one device than another. For example, men with impaired manual dexterity will do better with malleable or mechani-

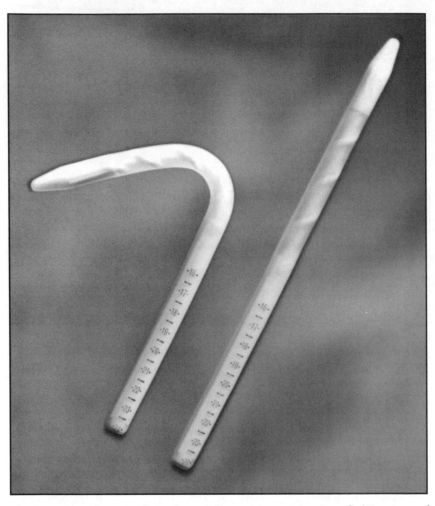

Figure 11-1: Semirigid penile prosthesis, Mentor Acu-Form®. (Courtesy of Mentor, Inc.)

cal devices than with inflatable devices. On the other hand, if repeated cystoscopy or transurethral procedures are expected (eg, in patients with bladder cancer), an inflatable device should be the preferred choice (Table 11-3).

Implantation Technique

For malleable prostheses, the most convenient incision is the penoscrotal incision, which facilitates corporeal dilation in difficult cases and, if perforation occurs, can be extended proximally or distally to correct the problem. For mechanical devices (Dura II™), the best incision is a distal semicircumcision or circumcision. For inflatable devices, several incisions have been used: (1) high, transverse scrotal incision; (2)

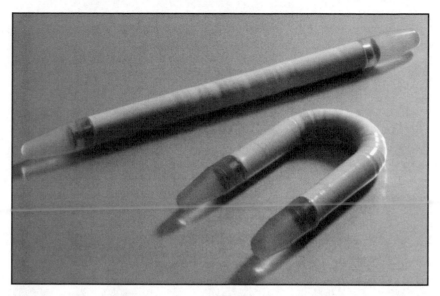

Figure 11-2: Duraphase® penile prosthesis. (Courtesy of Timm Medical.)

penoscrotal incision; and (3) suprapubic incision.

Longitudinal corporotomies about 2 cm long are made on each corpus cavernosum after stay sutures are placed. Dilation to 14 mm distally and 16 mm proximally is done with a Hegar's dilator or the metal rod used for corporeal length measurement. A sizing instrument is used, and the total

---

Table 11-1: Author's Indications and Contraindications for Implantation of Penile Prosthesis

Indications

- Failed or declined nonprosthetic therapies (oral PDE 5 inhibitor, intracavernous injection, transurethral therapy, or vacuum constriction device) in patients with organic erectile dysfunction

- Failed sex or psychosexual therapy and nonprosthetic therapies in patients with psychogenic erectile dysfunction

Contraindications

- Temporary or reversible impotence
- Unrealistic expectations
- Convicted sex offender
- Active venereal or infectious disease

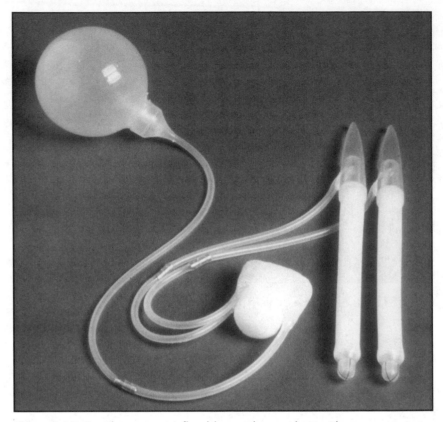

Figure 11-3: Three-piece inflatable penile prosthesis. The reservoir is implanted in the prevesical area, the cylinders within the corpora cavernosa, and the pump in the scrotal sac. (Courtesy of American Medical Systems, Inc.)

corporeal length is determined from the crus to the midglans.

The correct-length malleable or mechanical device is placed in the corpora cavernosa, and the wound is closed. For inflatable prostheses, the cylinder, pump, and reservoir are then filled with normal saline for implantation. The cylinders are implanted distally with the aid of the Furlow cylinder inserter. Any rear tip extenders are applied if needed, and the proximal cylinder is inserted into the proximal corpus cavernosum. The

wounds are closed with the help of a needle guard to avoid perforating the inflatable portion of the device. A dartos pouch is then created in the scrotum, and the pump is placed in it.

For reservoir implantation, a Foley catheter is inserted and the bladder is completely emptied. If surgery is through a suprapubic incision, the rectus sheath is separated and a prevesical space is created under direct vision to house the reservoir. If surgery is through penoscrotal or scrotal incision, long scissors are used to

Table 11-2: Penile Prostheses[1,2]

Type	Prosthesis	Vendor
Malleable	Acu-Form®	Mentor
	600M™/650M™	AMS
Mechanical	Dura II™	Timm Medical
Inflatable		
Two-piece	Ambicor®	AMS
Three-piece	Titan™ (3 connectors)	Mentor
	Alpha-1 (1 connector)	Mentor
	Alpha-1 (narrow base)	Mentor
	700 CX™	AMS
	700 CXM™	AMS
	700 Ultrex™ (3 connectors)	AMS
	700 Ultrex™ Plus (1 connector)	AMS

AMS = American Medical Systems

perforate the transversalis fascia in the floor of the external ring. The scissors are placed medial to the cord structures to avoid injury. A long-blade nasal speculum is then introduced into the fascial defect and holds this defect open as the empty reservoir is inserted into the retropubic space. The reservoir is filled with 65 mL or 100 mL of normal saline. The pump and the reservoir are connected with a sutureless connector. A suction drain is placed for overnight drainage before the subcutaneous layer and the skin are closed in layers.

Results

The malleable devices generally last longer than the inflatable ones. Patients should be informed that a 5% to 15% failure rate is expected in the first 5 years and that most devices will fail in 10 to 15 years and will need to be replaced.[3-6] Potential complications include mechanical failures, cylinder leaks, tubing leaks, infection,[7,8] perforation, persistent pain, and self-inflation.

Penile prosthesis implantation is ingenious, providing excellent re-

Table 11-3: Choosing the Right Penile Prosthesis

Profession or Conditions	Preferred Type of Prosthesis
Athletes, teachers, swimmers	Inflatable
History of bladder cancer or urinary stone	Inflatable
Prostatism or urethral stricture	Inflatable
Peyronie's disease	Avoid AMS Ultrex™
Small or fibrotic penis	AMS CXM™, Mentor Narrow Base
Poor manual dexterity	Semirigid, mechanical
High surgical risk	Semirigid, mechanical

sults and a high satisfaction rate. However, it is also a high-risk procedure and is fertile ground for litigation. Any complications resulting from implantation of penile prostheses, such as persistent pain, infection, or device failure, are potential excuses for legal action against the surgeon or the manufacturer. The risk of silicone is less a concern in penile prostheses because no silicone gel is used. However, infection of the prosthesis can result in severe scarring and penile shrinkage and can have a significant psychologic impact on the patient's ego and marriage. Therefore, an informed consent covering the following should be given to the patient before surgery: (1) a number of less invasive and highly effective alternative treatment options are available; (2) no penile prosthesis will achieve the length, girth, and flaccidity of the patient's natural erection; (3) the chance of infection is 3% to 5%, with the penis becoming much smaller and shorter if this occurs; and (4) all man-made devices, including penile pros-

thesis, eventually will fail, and, if so, surgery will be required to replace the device. The life expectancy of a prosthesis is 5 to 10 years, but it may fail before that time.

References

1. Mulcahy JJ: Overview of penile implants. In: Mulcahy JJ, ed. *Topics in Clinical Urology: Diagnosis and Management of Male Sexual Dysfunction.* New York, Igaku-Shoin, 1997, pp 218-230.

2. Montague DK, Lakin MM: Inflatable penis prostheses: the AMS 700 penile prosthesis. *Probl Urol* 1993;7:328-333.

3. Fallon B, Ghanem H: Sexual performance and satisfaction with penile prostheses in impotence of various etiologies. *Int J Impot Res* 1990;2:35-42.

4. Goldstein I, Bertero EB, Kaufman JM, et al: Early experience with the first pre-connected 3-piece inflatable penile prosthesis: the Mentor Alpha-1. *J Urol* 1993;150:1814-1818.

5. Krauss DJ, Lantinga LJ, Carey MP, et al: Use of the malleable penile prosthesis in the treatment of erectile dysfunction: a prospective study of postoperative adjustment. *J Urol* 1989;142:988-991.

6. Lewis RW: Long-term results of penile prosthetic implants. *Urol Clin North Am* 1995;22:847-856.

7. Wilson SK, Delk JR 2nd: Inflatable penile implant infection: predisposing factors and treatment suggestions. *J Urol* 1995;153:659-661.

8. Radomski SB, Herschorn S: Risk factors associated with penile prosthesis infection. *J Urol* 1992;147:383-385.

Chapter 12

Priapism

Priapism is persistent, painful erection of the penis, not accompanied by sexual stimulation or desire. Any erection persisting more than 6 hours should be considered priapism. Our animal studies showed that after this time, the intracavernous blood gases began to show ischemic changes. Transforming growth factor-β mRNA also expresses in the penile tissue after 6 hours.

Classification

Priapism can be classified into two types: ischemic (low-flow) and nonischemic (high-flow) priapism, as determined by intracavernous blood gases and penile blood flow studies.

Etiology

Many conditions can cause priapism. Some are secondary to diseases, medication, or injury, while many are without known causes and are termed *idiopathic* (Table 12-1).

History and Physical Examination

The diagnosis of priapism is usually based on history and physical examination. Priapism associated with intracavernous pharmacotherapy occurs more often in patients with neurogenic and psychogenic impotence, and the diagnosis is evident. Sickle cell priapism often occurs in teenagers, and recurrence is common. Acute low-flow (veno-occlusive) priapism, if lasting more than several hours, usually is painful because of changes associated with tissue ischemia. In contrast, most cases of high-flow (arterial) priapism are painless and usually follow perineal injury or direct injury to the penis.

On physical examination, the corpora cavernosa are fully rigid in low-flow priapism and partially to fully rigid in high-flow priapism. The glans and corpus spongiosum are not involved, except in rare cases of tricorporeal priapism. A thorough physical examination should include abdominal and neurologic examinations. Chronic priapism and acute intermittent (stuttering) priapism may be more difficult to diagnose because of atypical physical findings. Our management algorithm is illustrated in Figure 12-1.

Laboratory Testing

A blood sample should be obtained for hemoglobin S determination and to rule out leukemia. Urinalysis and urine culture also should be obtained

Table 12-1: Etiology of Priapism

High-flow Priapism
- Perineal or penile injury
- Light general anesthesia (neurogenic)

Low-flow Priapism
- Medication: anticoagulants, psychotropics, anticonvulsants, androgen
- Procedure: intracavernous injection of vasodilators, hyperalimentation
- Diseases: sickle cell disease or trait, leukemia, multiple myeloma, urinary tract inflammation or infection
- Neurologic: spinal injury
- Idiopathic

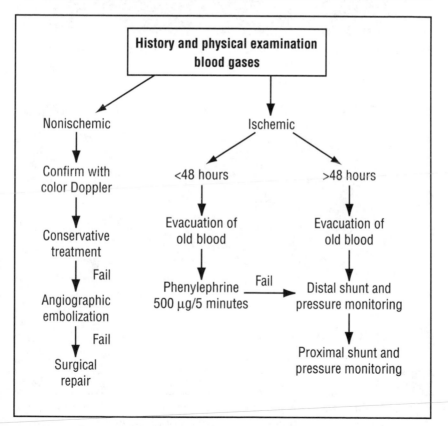

Figure 12-1: Treatment algorithm for priapism.

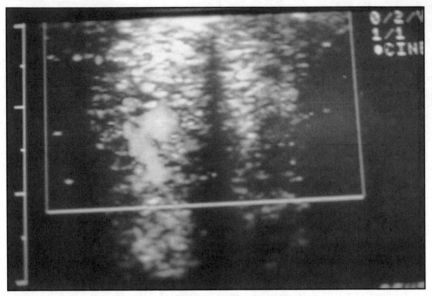

Figure 12-2: Color duplex ultrasound shows ruptured cavernous artery with pooling of blood within the corpus cavernosum in a patient with high-flow priapism after a straddle injury.

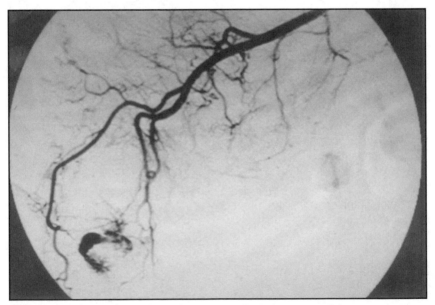

Figure 12-3: Selective internal pudendal arteriogram of the same patient shows ruptured cavernous artery with pooling of blood in the area of proximal corpus cavernosum.

Table 12-2: α-Adrenergic Agents for the Treatment of Priapism

Drug	Usual Dose
Epinephrine	10-20 µg
Phenylephrine	250-500 µg

After aspiration of 10 to 20 mL of blood, give intracavernous injection every 5 minutes until detumescence occurs.

to rule out urinary tract infection. Cavernous blood gas measurement is useful when the type of priapism needs to be determined: blood gas values similar to those of venous blood indicate low-flow disease; values similar to arterial blood suggest high-flow priapism. All cases of priapism begin as high-flow; therefore, cavernous blood gas measurement, if done early, may be misleading. Technetium (Tc) 99m scan has been advocated as a means of differentiating between the two types: uptake is high in arterial priapism and low in the veno-occlusive type.[1] We prefer blood gas determination and, if doubt exists, a color-coded duplex ultrasound scan of the cavernous arteries and the corpora cavernosa. No cavernous arterial flow with distended corpora cavernosa occurs in low-flow priapism, while a ruptured artery with unregulated blood pooling in the area of injury often occurs in trauma-induced high-flow priapism (Figures 12-2 and 12-3).

Nonsurgical Treatment of Priapism

Low-Flow Priapism

Treatment is aimed at the primary cause of priapism if it can be identified. The goals are to abort the erection, thereby preventing permanent damage to the corpora (which would lead to impotence), and to relieve pain. Medical management should always be tried before resorting to surgery. Ample evidence suggests that the risk of fibrosis and impotence increases with time. Generally, the incidence of impotence is less if erection is aborted within 24 hours.

Medical treatment. Medical treatment is aimed at decreasing arterial inflow and increasing venous outflow. The first line of treatment involves aspiration of the corpora and intracavernous injection of an α-adrenergic agonist (Table 12-2). Epinephrine, norepinephrine, and phenylephrine all have similar effects. We recommend initial aspiration of the corpora via a 21-gauge butterfly needle followed by injection of 250 to 500 µg phenylephrine, a pure α_1-adrenergic stimulant, every 5 minutes until detumescence takes place. The phenylephrine solution is made by mixing 10 mg/mL of phenylephrine with 19 mL of normal saline. Alternatively, oral terbutaline (Brethine®) 5 or 10 mg has been effective in inducing detumescence in some patients when priapism is related to intracavernous injection. A response rate of up to 36% has been reported in patients treated with terbutaline, compared with only 12% with placebo.[2]

Sickle cell disease. Sickle cell disorder accounts for approximately 28% of all cases of priapism; 42% of adults and 64% of children with sickle cell disease will eventually develop priapism. Although high-flow priapism in patients with sickle cell disease has recently been reported,[3] most cases are low flow. Treatment should be prompt and conservative because priapism often recurs in these patients. After ruling out other causes, the clinician should treat the patient with aggressive hydration, oxygenation, and metabolic alkalinization to reduce further sickling. Supertransfusion and erythropheresis should be second-line therapy. Aspiration and injection of diluted phenylephrine should be performed as soon as possible.

Recurrent priapism. Stuttering or recurrent priapism often occurs in patients with sickle cell trait or disease and in non-sickle cell patients with prior episodes. The mechanism is unknown, although alteration of adrenoceptors or scarring of intracavernous venules might be partially responsible. An oral α-adrenergic medication (eg, Entex® LA, one tablet b.i.d.) can be used for prevention. If not effective, an α-adrenergic agent such as phenylephrine (500 mg every 5 minutes until detumescence) can be self-injected. If sexual function is not a concern, an antiandrogen or a gonadotropin-releasing hormone agonist[4,5] (such as leuprolide acetate depot [Lupron Depot®] supension 7.5 mg/month for several months) that suppresses nocturnal penile erection can be helpful in preventing recurrence.

High-Flow Priapism

In the early stages, ice packing may cause vasospasm and spontaneous thrombosis of the ruptured artery. Three cases of spontaneous resolution have been observed by Ilkay and Levine that prompted them to propose conservative treatment of high-flow priapism.[6] However, most cases of delayed cavernous arterial rupture do not spontaneously subside, and arteriography with embolization of the internal pudendal artery usually is required.[7]

Complications of Medical Treatment

Untreated veno-occlusive priapism leads to corporeal fibrosis and impotence. Complications of treatment can be classified as early and late. Early complications include acute hypertension, headache, palpitations and cardiac arrhythmia from α-adrenergic agents, bleeding, infection, and urethral injury from needle puncture. Two deaths and one case of skin necrosis have been reported after injection of 2 mg to 4 mg of undiluted metaraminol (Aramine®).[8] Hematoma of the shaft after corporeal aspiration and irrigation is also common.

The most important late complications of priapism are fibrosis and impotence. Incidence is directly related to the duration of priapism and the aggressiveness of treatment. Although the overall impotence rate in low-flow priapism has been as high as 50% in the literature, almost all patients will regain their previous potency if the priapism is aborted by medical therapy within 12 to 24 hours. High-flow arterial priapism has a better prognosis, with a reported impotence rate of 0% to 20%.

Surgery for Ischemic Priapism

In ischemic priapism lasting more than 36 hours, we prefer to perform a

Table 12-3: Surgical Procedures for Ischemic Priapism

Distal Shunt		Proximal Shunt	
Ebbehoj	(1975)	Quackles	(1964)
Winter	(1976)	Odelowo	(1988)
Goulding	(1980)		
Datta	(1980)	**Cavernosum-Venous Shunt**	
Al-Ghorab	(1981)	Grayhack	(1964)
Hashmat	(1993)	Barry	(1976)
Kilinic	(1993)		

glans-cavernosum shunt with an 11-blade knife under regional or general anesthesia. The stagnant blood is milked out by hand, followed by irrigation with normal saline—not heparin solution—until the return is red. Monitoring the intracavernous pressure is useful in determining how many shunts are needed to provide adequate drainage and prevent recurrence. If the intracavernous pressure can be maintained below 40 mm Hg for 10 minutes after the skin incisions are closed, shunting should be successful.[9] In patients with severe edema or fibrosis of the distal penis, a proximal shunt will be needed. I prefer to perform spongiosocavernous shunt at the proximal portion of the urethral bulb. The surgical procedures are listed in Table 12-3.

Postoperative Management

After the shunting procedure, the corpora cavernosa are drained through the deep and superficial dorsal veins and corpus spongiosum. Circular compressive dressing should not be used because it may cut off all the draining systems of the corpus cavernosa and result in further ischemia and tissue necrosis.

Perioperative antibiotics should be given to all patients with ischemic priapism to prevent infection of the ischemic tissue. Catheters should be removed as soon as possible.

Postoperative Complications

Early complications include recurrence of priapism, bleeding, infection, skin necrosis, abscess, cellulitis, gangrene, urethral damage, urethrocutaneous fistula, and urethral stricture. Late complications include fibrosis of erectile tissue, impotence, and failure of venous shunt to close spontaneously, leading to impotence. The risk of postoperative infection must be anticipated, and adequate perioperative antibiotics must be administered. The most frequent complication of sickle cell priapism is recurrence.

Patients with prolonged or repetitive episodes of priapism are likely to suffer erectile dysfunction after resolution of their condition (secondary to fibrosis). In most reports, postoperative potency is about 50%. Traumatic priapism seems to have the best prognosis. Treatment of nonischemic priapism by selective pudendal artery embolization has the best success in preserving potency.

Surgery for Nonischemic Priapism

If priapism persists after several months of watchful waiting, angiographic embolization of the ruptured artery should be performed.[10] If embolization is not successful, surgical exploration and ligation of the ruptured artery are indicated.

Informed Consent

About 50% of patients develop some degree of erectile dysfunction, regardless of the method of management. Therefore, a carefully worded informed consent explaining that impotence may result should be read to the patient. The patient or one of his relatives then should sign it with an appropriate witness. This is an area of high medicolegal interest.

Conclusion

Priapism is uncommon, and low-flow priapism is a urologic emergency. Almost all cases can be successfully aborted with injection of a diluted α-adrenergic agonist if treatment begins within 12 hours of onset. Tissue damage can thus be prevented and potency preserved. High-flow priapism itself does not cause erectile tissue damage, but injury to the erectile tissue and nerves from perineal trauma may be associated with delayed recovery of potency after treatment. The best diagnostic tool is a color-coded duplex ultrasonogram, and angiographic embolization is the treatment of choice, if watchful waiting fails.

References

1.   Hashmat AI, Raju S, Singh I, et al: 99mTc penile scan: an investigative modality in priapism. *Urol Radiol* 1989; 11:58-60.

2.   Lowe FC, Jarow JP: Placebo-controlled study of oral terbutaline and pseudoephedrine in management of prostaglandin E_1-induced prolonged erections. *Urology* 1993;42:51-54.

3.   Ramos CE, Park JS, Ritchey ML, et al: High flow priapism associated with sickle cell disease. *J Urol* 1995;153:1619-1621.

4.   Levine LA, Guss SP: Gonadotropin-releasing hormone analogues in the treatment of sickle cell anemia-associated priapism. *J Urol* 1993;150:475-477.

5.   Steinberg J, Eyre RC: Management of recurrent priapism with epinephrine self-injection and gonadotropin-releasing hormone analogue. *J Urol* 1995;153:152-153.

6.   Ilkay AK, Levine LA: Conservative management of high-flow priapism. *Urology* 1995;46:419-424.

7.   Brock G, Breza J, Lue TF, et al: High flow priapism: a spectrum of disease. *J Urol* 1993;150:968-971.

8.   Bondil P, Guionie R: Prolonged drug-induced erection. Treatment and prevention. *Ann Urol (Paris)* 1988;22:411-415.

9.   Lue TF, Hellstrom WJ, McAninch JW, et al: Priapism: a refined approach to diagnosis and treatment. *J Urol* 1986; 136:104-108.

10.   Walker TG, Grant PW, Goldstein I, et al: 'High-flow' priapism: treatment with superselective transcatheter embolization. *Radiology* 1990;174:1053-1054.

Chapter 13

Peyronie's Disease

P eyronie's disease was first reported as *indurato penis plastica* in 1743 by Francois Gigot de la Peyronie, surgeon to King Louis XV of France. The disease has since borne his name. Peyronie's disease is a localized connective tissue disorder that primarily affects the tunica albuginea and the areolar space between the tunica albuginea and erectile tissue. It is characterized by the development of a circumscribed, painless, dense, fibrous plaque, resulting in angulation of the erect penis. The damage to the patient's self-esteem and disruption of his personal life can make it a physically and psychologically debilitating disease.

Presentation

Reports indicate that as many as 3% of adult men are affected by Peyronie's disease. Most cases are in white men, usually during the 5th and 6th decades of life, but reports have identified the disease in teens and octogenarians. Peyronie's disease has two discernible phases: acute and chronic.

The acute phase is characterized by a triad of symptoms: plaque, pain, and penile deformity. Pain is most pronounced during erection and is present in 30% to 40% of patients. This phase normally lasts several months; during this period, pain gradually subsides while the plaque becomes harder and penile deformity becomes more pronounced. The chronic phase is represented by another triad of symptoms: plaque, deformity, and erectile dysfunction.[1]

Natural History

Gelbard et al found that some resolution of the disease occurred in 13% of patients, gradual progression occurred in 40%, and 47% of the patients showed no change.[1] Complete resolution is rare and often takes several years. Prognosis is good when the patient is young and has a soft plaque (<2 cm) and when the duration of symptoms is brief. Penile deformity usually persists in patients with substantial early penile angulation (>45°). Moreover, prognosis is poor when calcification develops within the plaque.

Peyronie's Disease and Impotence

Most patients retain the ability to obtain and maintain erection. However, they may have difficulties in vaginal penetration and sexual activ-

Table 13-1: Proposed Causes of Peyronie's Disease

Medical: venereal disease, arteriosclerosis, diabetes mellitus, phlebitis

Pharmacologic: barbiturates, β-blockers, vitamin E deficiency

Familial: associated with Dupuytren's contracture of hands

Traumatic: sexual excess, delamination injury

Autoimmune: altered response to vascular trauma

ity resulting from curvature, pain on intromission, or partner dyspareunia.

Inadequate erection may occur in about 20% of patients with symptomatic Peyronie's disease. Vascular disease, either arterial or veno-occlusive dysfunction, has been reported in as many as 70% of men who have erectile dysfunction. About 36% of impotent men with Peyronie's disease had abnormal arterial blood flow, and 59% had evidence of veno-occlusive dysfunction. Therefore, vascular insufficiency associated with Peyronie's disease is key in impotence.[2,3] Plaque-induced or site-specific venous leaks during cavernosography in Peyronie's disease and in patients with blunt penile trauma have also been reported.[4]

Distal penile flaccidity may be the main problem that precludes vaginal penetration. This can result from concomitant vascular insufficiency or the constrictive effects of plaque on the penis. A duplex color ultrasound study after intracavernous injection of a vasodilator usually identifies the cause.

Causes and Pathogenesis

Many diseases, medications, and conditions have been proposed as causes of Peyronie's disease, but none has been proven (Table 13-1).

Vande Berg et al suggested that Peyronie's disease is an autoimmune response to vascular trauma.[5] Several recent studies also showed features of autoimmunity, particularly the cell-mediated response.[6] Stewart et al showed that antibodies to elastin are present, as are increased serum levels of antitropoelastin (reflecting elastin synthesis) and anti-α-elastin (reflecting elastin destruction) in all patients with Peyronie's disease.[7]

Although a familial tendency toward Peyronie's disease has been proposed, data conflict over the association of HLA-B27 or HLA-B7 with the disease.[8] The disease is also associated with other fibromatosis of the elastic tissue. About 10% of Peyronie's patients have Dupuytren's contracture; however, the coincidence of Peyronie's disease in patients with Dupuytren's disease is approximately 3%. In addition, plantar fibrosis and tympanosclerosis occur in patients with Peyronie's disease but are rare.

Regulation of collagen synthesis by many endogenous and exogenous factors, especially producers of oxygen-free radicals such as ascorbic acid and other biologically active peptides such as epidermal growth factor (EGF) and insulin-like growth factor (IGF), has been reported in the pathogenesis of

Peyronie's disease. Transforming growth factor-beta (TGF-β) has recently attracted much interest as a cytokine that affects the deposition of extracellular matrix and induces fibrosis in the tunica albuginea.[9,10]

The most widely accepted theory has been proposed by Devine and Horton.[11] They hypothesize that Peyronie's disease is caused by an abnormal fibrotic reaction to minimal trauma. The tunica is a laminated structure, with outer longitudinal and inner circular layers. The latter fuse in the midline to form the septum. Bending of the partially rigid penis may delaminate the tunica in the area of stress and cause microvascular trauma. Destabilization of the axial erectile rigidity mechanism, which may occur in a partially rigid penis, is a potential risk for buckling injury.[12,13]

This process leads to inflammation and induration with deposition of nonpolarized collagen. Over the next 6 to 9 months, remodeling causes some polarization of collagen fibers, and eventual scarring occurs in susceptible patients. The inflammation is literally 'trapped' for several months, resulting in release of large amounts of cytokines, destruction of elastic fibers, and overproduction of collagens. The ultrastructural findings by transmission and scanning electron microscopy show that in normal tunica albuginea, elastic fibers form an irregular lattice network on which the collagen fibrils lie. The multilayered nature of the tunica appears to be distinct and able to slide on the adjacent layers. In this way, flexibility is achieved. In Peyronie's plaques, collagen fibers are immature and densely and irregularly packed,

resulting in focal loss of elasticity. The affected area of the tunica albuginea does not expand on erection and, therefore, causes curvature, indentation, or shortening of the penis.[14,15]

Differential Diagnosis

Although the diagnosis of Peyronie's disease is fairly straightforward, a sarcoma, though rare, may be confused with Peyronie's disease. This possibility must be ruled out with a biopsy, especially when the plaque has grown rapidly. When evaluating patients with Peyronie's disease, many other causes of bending and induration of the penis also must be considered, including congenital curvature of the penis, chordee with or without hypospadias, penile dorsal artery thrombosis, fibrosis secondary to local trauma, leukemic infiltration of the corpora cavernosa, ventral curvature secondary to urethral stricture disease, benign or malignant primary or secondary tumors, late syphilitic lesion, or penile infiltration with lymphogranuloma venereum.

Diagnosis

The diagnosis of Peyronie's disease usually is apparent by the patient history and physical examination of the penis.

Medical and Psychosexual History

The medical history should include time and mode of onset (sudden or gradual), course of disease (stable or progressive), history of penile surgery or trauma, medication or drug abuse, and family history of Peyronie's disease or Dupuytren's contracture.

A detailed psychosexual history also should be sought. This includes

Table 13-2: Common Agents for Peyronie's Disease

Oral	Dose	Action	Success*	Side Effects
Vitamin E	800 IU/d	Enhances vasodilation and inhibits platelet aggregation; antioxidant	0%-91%	None
Amino-benzoate potassium (Potaba®)	12 mg/d	Increases oxygen utilization at the tissue level; enhances the enzyme MAO activity, which decreases serotonin effect	16%-88%	Stomach upset (32 tablets/d)
Procarbazine (Matulane®)	100 mg/d	Cytotoxic agent; MAO inhibitor	10%-56%	Leukopenia, thrombocy-topenia, GI upset, germinal epithelial damage
Tamoxifen (Nolvadex®)	40 mg/d	Increases the secretion of TGF-β, (?) which decreases the inflammatory response and fibrogenesis	55%	Reduced libido, facial flushing, reduced ejaculatory volume
Colchicine	2.4 mg/d	Antitubulin; decreases collagen synthesis and induces collagenase activity	37%-78%	Diarrhea, stomach upset, bone marrow suppression

MAO = monoamine oxidase, TGF-β = transforming growth factor-β, GI = gastrointestinal
*Reduction of curvature or size of plaque; not pain relief

penile rigidity during erection, shortening, induration, hourglass constriction, or pain with or without erection. Other important information also should be determined, such as ability to have intercourse, adequacy of erection (rigidity and duration), frequency of intercourse, libido, and psychological impact. A photograph of the patient's erect penis to identify the

Table 13-3: Common Intralesional Therapy for Peyronie's Disease

Intralesional	Dose	Action	Success	Side Effects
Cortisone	25 mg/ week	Anti-inflammatory	30%	Tissue atrophy and scarring; decreased chance of successful surgery
Collagenase	6,000-14,000 units	Purified bacterial enzyme that selectively dissolves collagen	36%	Pain, tunical tear, ecchymosis
Orgotein	4 mg/ 2 weeks	Anti-inflammatory with pronounced superoxide dismutase activity	50%	None
Interferon-α	1,000,000 units/ week	Inhibits proliferation and collagen production	5%-25%	Myalgia, fever
Verapamil	10 mg/ 2 weeks	Calcium-channel blocker, antifibrosis	0%-85%	Ecchymosis, hematoma, sensation change (temporary)

extent, direction, and character of erectile distortion is helpful.

Physical Examination

Examination of the penis in patients with Peyronie's disease is facilitated by the gentle stretching of the penis. This helps determine the size and location of plaques. The patient should also be examined for the presence of Dupuytren's and plantar fascial contractures. Further diagnostic studies should include photography or drawing of the erect penis after intracavernous injection or vacuum erection device.

Other Investigations

High-resolution superficial sonography allows for detailed objective assessment of the plaque and calcification, as well as for detection of multiple areas of involvement. Sonography can also be used to assess plaque before and after medical therapy or surgery. Therefore, sonography is the most objective means of assessing plaque dimensions at any stage of the disease. Color duplex ultrasonography after intracavernous injection of a vasodilator can help assess penile vascular function.[2,16] This technique can also be used to identify collateral arterial connections between the dorsal and cavernous as well as the cavernous and spongiosal arteries; injury to these collateral arteries during surgery for Peyronie's disease may cause postoperative impotence.

In patients in whom venous leak is suspected, a pharmacologic cavernosometry and cavernosography may help determine the degree and sites of venous leak.

Management
Nonsurgical Treatment

Many treatments have been proposed for Peyronie's disease. In 1743, de la Peyronie recommended bathing in the Barege spa. Many agents have been used to treat Peyronie's disease, with varying rates of success (Tables 13-2 and 13-3). Oral agents include vitamin E, aminobenzoate potassium (Potaba®), procarbazine (Matulane®), tamoxifen (Nolvadex®), corticosteroids, and colchicine. Topical application of iodine, mercury, iodoform, and camphor has also been reported. Intra-lesional injection of parathyroid hormone, dimethyl sulfoxide, cortisone, collagenase, orgotein, interferon, and verapamil has been used with some success.[17,18] Other modalities of treatment, such as radiotherapy, ultrasound, and laser, have also been reported.[19]

It is difficult to assess the value of treatment without a randomized, placebo-controlled, large-scale clinical study. Nonsurgical treatment will continue to evolve, and new agents and modalities will be introduced until more effective treatment options are proven by clinical trials and accepted by the medical community.

Surgical Treatment
Nonprosthetic surgery. Tunica shortening procedures have been used for a long time with high success. Plication of the tunica[20] and Nesbit's wedge resection are the most popular techniques. Incision or wedge resection of the tunica requires dissection of the neurovascular bundle or the corpus spongiosum. The surgeon then places absorbable sutures to shorten the longer side of the tunica. Many researchers have reported that this is a relatively simple, safe, and effective procedure. Modifications of this technique were reported as an effective alternative to the original.[21,22] Because absorbable sutures are used, we have seen several penile herniations because of dehiscence of the tunica.

We prefer performing plication under local anesthesia, after erection is produced by intracavernous injection of papaverine or alprostadil. For ventral curvature, two to three pairs of nonabsorbable sutures (2-0 Ticron or Tevdex) are placed between the deep dorsal vein and the dorsal arteries. For dorsal curvature, the same sutures are placed in the paraurethral ridges. No dissection of the neurovascular bundle or corpus spongiosum is necessary. Because the procedure is performed on an erect penis and the sutures are tied until the penis is straight, this is the least invasive and most successful technique (Figure 13-1).

Lengthening of the tunica with graft replacement is indicated in severe shortening or hourglass deformity of the penis. Many autologous tissue (eg, dermis, temporalis fascia, dura mater, tunica vaginalis, dorsal or saphenous vein), cadaveric material

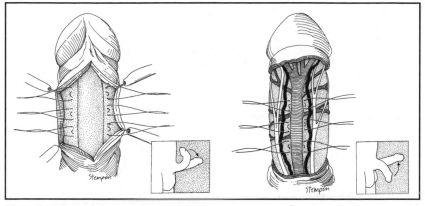

Figure 13-1: (a) Perispongiosal plication sutures for dorsal curvature. (b) Sutures between dorsal vein and dorsal arteries for ventral curvature.

(lyophized human pericardium, porcine small intestine submucosa), and synthetic materials (Dacron and Gore-Tex®) have been used with different results. Excision of the plaque, with the intent of removing all the diseased tunica, has long been the standard approach. However, we now believe it is unnecessary because the pathologic process of Peyronie's disease extends far beyond the plaque, and removing a large area of tunica albuginea requires a large graft that may further impair erectile function. In 1991, Gelbard and Hayden proposed plaque incision and grafting rather than excision.[23] This is gradually becoming more popular.

No graft material is perfect for replacing the diseased tunica albuginea. The synthetic material, dura, and fascia may provide a strong covering for the tunica; however, they do not stretch as much as the normal tunica, and curvature may recur after the graft is fixed to the surrounding tissue. Synthetic material also has some risk of foreign body reaction and infection. Dermis is a good substitute and plentiful, but it tends to contract after several months,

causing recurrence. We prefer saphenous vein graft because (1) it regains blood supply within minutes; (2) the endothelium limits permeation of blood and therefore does not cause hematoma above the graft site; and (3) its smooth-muscle coat reacts to high pressure in the penis and becomes thicker and stronger in about 3 months. We have seen no recurrences at the graft site (Figure 13-2).

Postoperative erectile dysfunction after graft placement is a significant concern. Many reports have documented that erectile dysfunction may occur in up to 70% of patients. Several causes are possible: (1) concomitant vascular disease, (2) venous leak from graft failure, (3) fibrosis under or near the graft site, (4) arterial injury, and (5) nerve damage. We believe that most of these causes are preventable. For example, a preoperative color ultrasound can identify collateral circulation between the dorsal and cavernous arteries and thus prevent inadvertent injury. Dissection of the neurovascular bundle should always be performed under magnification to spare nerve fibers.

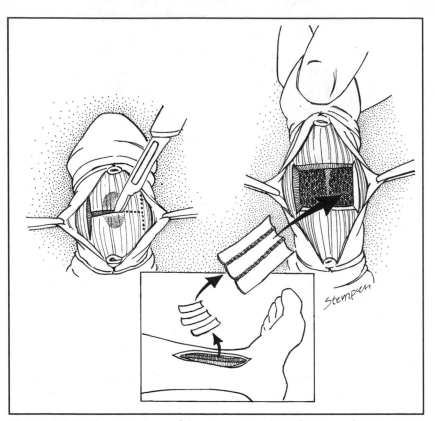

Figure 13-2: The main steps of the venous patch graft surgery for correction of penile deformity. Note the H-shaped incision of the tunica albuginea and use of the lower saphenous vein as graft material.

Proper handling of the graft can also prevent graft failure.

Penile prosthesis with or without grafting. In the past, if a patient had penile deformity and erectile dysfunction, he was automatically recommended for insertion of penile prosthesis. However, this indication has been modified since the less invasive treatments (eg, phosphodiesterase type 5 [PDE 5] inhibitors, intracavernous injection, intraurethral medication, vacuum constriction devices) replaced penile prosthesis as initial treatment. Many urologists

now offer reconstructive procedures to the patient if he responds well to any nonsurgical treatments for impotence. If the patient does not respond to these less invasive treatments, then penile prosthesis is offered.[24]

In most patients with mild to moderate deformity, insertion of a penile prosthesis tends to straighten the penis, and no additional procedure is necessary. However, if severe deformity still persists after the prosthesis is inflated, the surgeon can incise the plaque and cover the defect with a synthetic material such

Table 13-4: Complications of Surgery for Peyronie's Disease

Plication

- Hematoma
- Recurrent plaque
- Sensation change—from circumcision
- Persistent pain for more than 6 months

Venous Grafting

- Decreased penile sensation
- Persistent pain for more than 6 months
- Decreased penile rigidity
- Residual curvature or narrowing
- Recurrent plaque
- Wound infection

Penile Prosthesis

- Residual curvature (especially with Ultrex™ prosthesis)
- Infection
- Device failure
- Urinary difficulty

as Gore-Tex® or rectus sheath. Some propose a 'modeling' technique to forcefully bend the penis after the device is inflated to straighten the penis. Caution should be exercised during the maneuver because one patient has been reported to develop complete anesthesia of the penis after this procedure.

If an inflatable penile prosthesis is used, the distally expanding prostheses (eg, Ultrex™) are not recommended because, as the device lengthens, it also tends to bend the penis. The girth-expansion-only devices (eg, CX™, Alpha-1) are better choices in patients with penile curvature. Table 13-4 outlines the complications of surgical treatment for Peyronie's disease.

Peyronie's disease is one of the least understood diseases in urology. The pathogenesis is still not certain, the medical treatments are unpredictable and effective in less than 50% of patients, and controversies still exist about surgical approach. Several new research developments have shed some light on pathogenesis, which hopefully will improve our understanding and management for patients with this frustrating disease.

References

1. Gelbard MK, Dorey F, James K: The natural history of Peyronie's disease. *J Urol* 1990;144:1376-1379.

2. Levine LA, Coogan CL: Penile vascular assessment using color duplex sonography in men with Peyronie's disease. *J Urol* 1996;155:1270-1273.

3. Weidner W, Schroeder-Printzen I, Weiske WH, et al: Sexual dysfunction in Peyronie's disease: an analysis of 222 patients without previous local plaque therapy. *J Urol* 1997;157:325-328.

4. Penson DF, Seftel AD, Krane RJ, et al: The hemodynamic pathophysiology of impotence following blunt trauma to the erect penis. *J Urol* 1992;148:1171-1180.

5. Vande Berg JS, Devine CJ Jr, Horton CE, et al: Mechanisms of calcification in Peyronie's disease. *J Urol* 1982;127:52-54.

6. Ralph DJ, Mirakian R, Pryor JP, et al: The immunological features of Peyronie's disease. *J Urol* 1996;155:159-162.

7. Stewart S, Malto M, Sandberg L, et al: Increased serum levels of anti-elastin antibodies in patients with Peyronie's disease. *J Urol* 1994;152:105-106.

8. Leffell MS: Is there an immunogenetic basis for Peyronie's disease? *J Urol* 1997;157:295-297.

9. El-Sakka AI, Hassoba HM, Pillarisetty RJ, et al: Peyronie's disease is associated with an increase in transforming growth factor-beta protein expression. *J Urol* 1997;158:1391-1394.

10. El-Sakka AI, Hassoba HM, Chui RM, et al: An animal model of Peyronie's-like condition associated with an increase of transforming growth factor beta mRNA and protein expression. *J Urol* 1997; 158:2284-2290.

11. Devine CJ Jr, Horton CE: Peyronie's disease. *Clin Plast Surg* 1988;15:405-409.

12. Devine CJ Jr: International Conference on Peyronie's disease advances in basic and clinical research. March 17-19, 1993. Introduction. *J Urol* 1997;157:272-275.

13. Somers KD, Dawson DM: Fibrin deposition in Peyronie's disease plaque. *J Urol* 1997;157:311-315.

14. Akkus E, Carrier S, Baba K, et al: Structural alterations in the tunica albuginea of the penis: impact of Peyronie's disease, ageing and impotence. *Br J Urol* 1997;79:47-53.

15. Brock G, Hsu GL, Nunes L, et al: The anatomy of the tunica albuginea in the normal penis and Peyronie's disease. *J Urol* 1997;157:276-281.

16. Lopez JA, Jarow JP: Penile vascular evaluation of men with Peyronie's disease. *J Urol* 1993;149:53-55.

17. Wegner HE, Andresen R, Knispel HH, et al: Local interferon-alpha 2b is not an effective treatment in early-stage Peyronie's disease. *Eur Urol* 1997; 32:190-193.

18. Levine LA: Treatment of Peyronie's disease with intralesional verapamil injection. *J Urol* 1997;158:1395-1399.

19. Chevallier D, Benizri E, Volpe P, et al: La Peyronie disease. Historical, epidemiological, physiopathological data. Diagnostic and therapeutic approaches. *Rev Med Interne* 1997;18:41S-45S.

20. Nooter RI, Bosch JL, Schroder FH: Peyronie's disease and congenital penile curvature: long-term results of operative treatment with the plication procedure. *Br J Urol* 1994;74:497-500.

21. Rehman J, Benet A, Minsky LS, et al: Results of surgical treatment for abnormal penile curvature: Peyronie's disease and congenital deviation by modified Nesbit plication (tunical shaving and plication). *J Urol* 1997;157:1288-1291.

22. Licht MR, Lewis RW: Modified Nesbit procedure for the treatment of Peyronie's disease: a comparative outcome analysis. *J Urol* 1997;158:460-463.

23. Gelbard MK, Hayden B: Expanding contractures of the tunica albuginea due to Peyronie's disease with temporalis fascia free grafts. *J Urol* 1991;145:772-776.

24. Daitch JA, Angermeier KW, Lakin MM, et al: Long-term mechanical reliability of AMS 700 series inflatable penile prostheses: comparison of CX/CXM and Ultrex cylinders. *J Urol* 1997;158:1400-1402.

Chapter 14

Case Management Examples

Blessed is the man who, having nothing to say, abstains from giving wordy evidence of the fact.—George Eliot (1819-1880) (This is why algorithms are used in this chapter.)

Case Report 1

A 60-year-old musician with a 6-year history of hypertension and intermittent claudication complained of his inability to maintain an erection in the past year, though retaining normal sex drive and orgasm. History revealed that he was taking diuretics for hypertension and simvastatin (Zocor®) for high cholesterol. He had been smoking about one pack of cigarettes a day for 30 years and drank one glass of wine a day (Figure 14-1).

Based on the history, the underlying cause for this patient's erectile problem is likely to be vascular insufficiency. Extensive vascular work-up is not necessary (duplex ultrasound is optional if the patient wishes to know the degree of vascular insufficiency) because vascular surgery for these patients does not have a good success rate. If the less invasive treatments, such as oral agents, intracavernous injection, transurethral therapy, or vacuum constriction devices, are ineffective, then implantation of a penile prosthesis would be the best solution for this patient. As indicated in the algorithm, other tests, including neurologic and psychological testing, are not necessary because the history and physical examination do not suggest psychological or neurologic problems.

Case Report 2

A 28-year-old computer programmer complained of his inability to achieve a full erection since an automobile accident 3 years ago. He sustained a pelvic fracture and membranous urethral injury and underwent a urethroplasty 6 months later. He has been unable to have sexual intercourse since the accident and has not improved since the surgery (Figure 14-2).

The work-up in this algorithm is much more extensive for two reasons. First, the patient was involved in a car collision and sustained significant injury. Litigation among those involved in the accident is always a possibility and, therefore, a RigiScan® study is indicated to rule out malingering. Second, a pelvic or proximal urethral injury can cause neurogenic, vascular, or cavernous damage. If the injury is to the internal pudendal artery, proven by pharmacologic arteriography, arterial bypass surgery can have a high success rate (about 75%). Severe injury to the base of the penis can also cause fibrosis and venous leak. If the

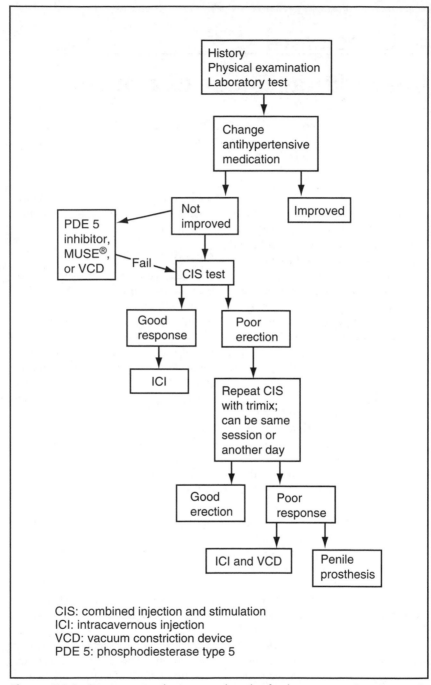

Figure 14-1: Diagnostic and treatment algorithm for the patient in Case Report 1.

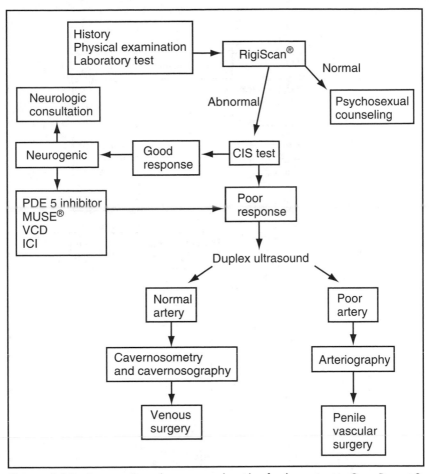

Figure 14-2: Diagnostic and treatment algorithm for the patient in Case Report 2.

cavernosography reveals a localized crural leak, surgical repair (crural ligation) can be curative.

Case Report 3

A 60-year-old teacher with a 10-year history of adult-onset diabetes mellitus, whose wife of 35 years died of cervical cancer 10 months ago, complained of low libido and an inability to get a solid erection since his wife's death (Figure 14-3).

Low sexual drive for this man can be psychologic as a result of his sorrow over the loss of his wife. It can also occur because of hypogonadism associated with long-term diabetes. Impotence can also be caused by vascular or neurologic complications from long-term diabetes. Again, this is not a good case for penile revascularization, and, therefore, extensive vascular work-up is not necessary. If the less invasive treatments are not

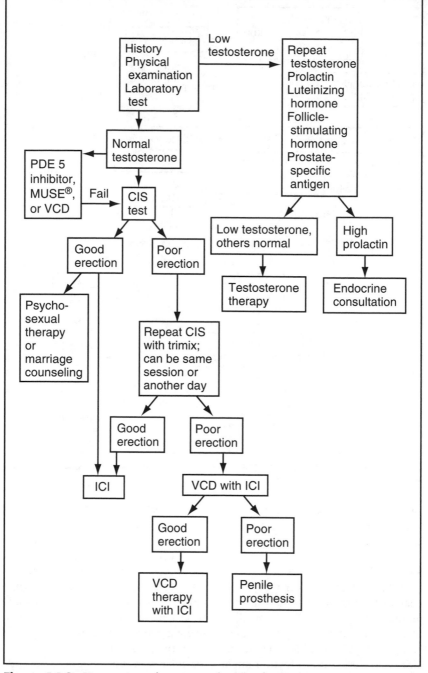

Figure 14-3: Diagnostic and treatment algorithm for the patient in Case Report 3.

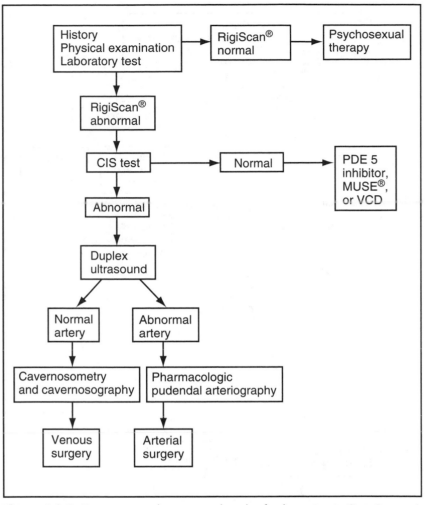

Figure 14-4: Diagnostic and treatment algorithm for the patient in Case Report 4.

effective, implantation of a penile prosthesis can be considered.

Case Report 4

A 22-year-old college student complained of his inability to achieve and maintain a rigid erection for as long as he could remember. He is in otherwise perfect health and is not a drug abuser. He recalled a bicycle accident with injury to his perineum when he was 10 years old (Figure 14-4).

This is a patient with primary impotence. Because psychological factors or ignorance may be significantly involved in this kind of case, a RigiScan® study should be performed to confirm or rule out psychogenic impotence. If the impotence is caused by misinformation or performance anxi-

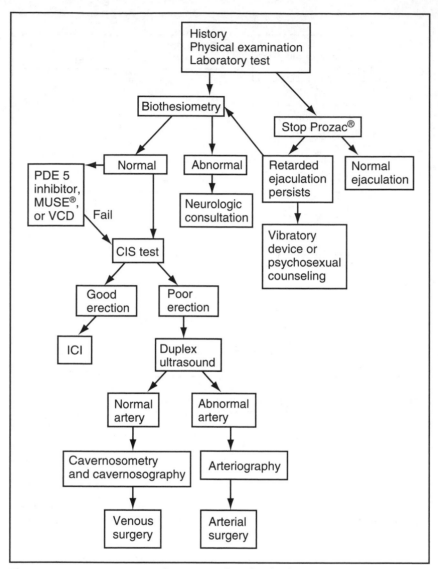

Figure 14-5: Diagnostic and treatment algorithm for the patient in Case Report 5.

ety, psychosexual therapy can be curative. On the other hand, a number of these patients do have congenital anomalies or injuries during childhood, and detailed examination and testing is indicated if RigiScan® results are abnormal. Vascular surgery does have a high success rate for young patients with congenital or acquired vascular insufficiency.

Case Report 5

A 40-year-old coast-to-coast truck driver complained of increasing difficulty in maintaining erection and achieving orgasm. He is taking fluoxetine (Prozac®) for mild depression. He also complained of intermittent back pain and numbness in his right leg off and on since sustaining a minor back injury 2 years ago (Figure 14-5).

Difficult ejaculation and orgasm are known side effects of fluoxetine and other serotonin reuptake inhibitors such as sertraline (Zoloft®) and clomipramine (Anafranil®); stopping fluoxetine may help his ejaculation. Interestingly, these side effects can turn into blessings for patients with premature ejaculation, and physicians have prescribed this group of medications with some success. This particular patient also gave a history of back injury that could result in disk herniation and nerve compression. Therefore, a more detailed neurologic examination by a neurologist is indicated. On the other hand, minor perineal injury can also occur from prolonged compression of the perineum and penile base. Because of his young age and health, he is a good candidate for vascular surgery if vascular testing reveals localized arterial insufficiency.

Index

A

α-adrenergic agonists 23, 129, 132

α-adrenergic blockers 22, 77, 92

abdominoperineal resection 30, 31, 47

acetylcholine 17, 19, 20, 37

acromegaly 56

Actis® 96

adenoma 32, 76

adenylate cyclase 22

adrenal failure 57

aging 6, 26, 28, 31, 33, 35, 36, 40, 41, 76, 117

AIDS 31, 40

alcohol 38, 39, 47, 54, 71, 91, 106

alcoholism 30, 31, 39, 40

Aldactone® 37

Aldomet® 37, 77

alkaloids 22

allergic contact dermatitis 74

Alpha-1 141

alpha-cyclodextrin 104

alprostadil (Caverject®, prostaglandin E₁) 30, 77, 96, 103-107, 138

alprostadil alfadex (Edex™) 104

Alprostadil Medicated Urethral System for Erection (MUSE®) 81, 84, 86, 87, 89, 90, 96, 98, 144-148

Alzheimer's disease 30

aminobenzoate potassium (Potaba®) 138

amoxapine 34

AMS 600M™/650M™ 123

AMS 700 CX™ 119, 123

AMS 700 CXM™ 119, 123

AMS 700 Ultrex™ 119, 123

AMS 700 Ultrex™ Plus 119, 123

AMS Ambicor® 119, 123

AMS Parylene™ 119

amyloidosis 31

Anabolic Steroids Control Act 74

Anafranil® 149

anatomic abnormalities 45

Androderm® 73-75

AndroGel® 74

androgen 32, 33, 40, 57, 73-76, 127

Android® 75

andropause 76

anemia 49

angina 41, 96

angiotensin-converting enzyme (ACE) 77

anti-α-elastin 134

antiandrogen 39, 54, 130

antibiotics 131